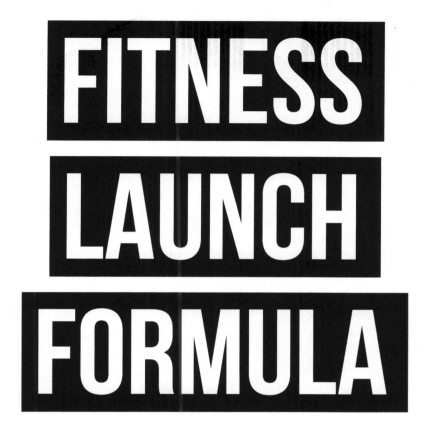

FITNESS LAUNCH FORMULA

The no fear, no b.s., no hype, action plan for launching a profitable fitness business in 60 days - from someone who's done it.

BRIAN DEVLIN

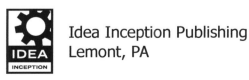
Idea Inception Publishing
Lemont, PA

COPYRIGHT

FITNESS LAUNCH FORMULA: The no fear, no b.s., no hype, action plan for launching a profitable fitness business in 60 days or less – from someone who's done it.

Brian Devlin
Idea Inception Publishing
Box 411
Lemont, PA 16851

Copyright 2012 by Brian Devlin & Idea Inception Publishing. Printed and bound in The USA.

Find us on the web at: IdeaInception.com.

To report errors, please send a note or screenshot to: support@fitproevolution.com

Idea Inception Publishing, a division of Fit Pro Evolution Inc.

Project Editor: Doug Williams

Book Designer and Author: Brian Devlin

Cover design, Illustration: Alexa I. Stefanou

ISBN: 978-0-9864256-0-8   Library of Congress Control Number: 2015901042

Don't Miss Your 2 Invaluable
Free Bonus Videos and Start Up Cheat Sheet!

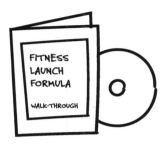 A personal walk-through video covering all the steps of the fitness launch formula

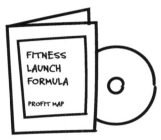 An in-depth and invaluable training video showing how to get your business to profit in month 1

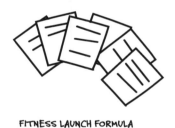 The fitness launch cheat sheets outlining all the steps of my formula

FITNESS LAUNCH FORMULA
CHEAT SHEETS

Congratulations, and thank you for investing in my book Fitness Launch Formula! Please don't forget to download your $297 bonus training package that I have included with your purchase.

This FREE training will really help you implement the strategies and tactics I discuss in the book quickly and efficiently. To grab your bonuses, simply go to www. FitProEvolution.com/flf-book-bonus/

Just my way of saying "thank you" for investing in my book!

CONTENTS

ACKNOWLEDGMENT

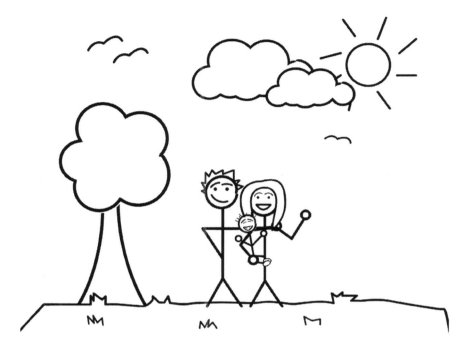

This book is dedicated to my beautiful wife Kim and our precious daughter Charli.

Thank you for giving me the encouragement and inspiration I needed to finally share my message with the world. You have been so supportive and kept me going on those days I just wanted to quit.

I thank God for allowing our paths to cross and allowing me to marry such an amazing woman. Together we will do great things.

INTRODUCTION

Imagine owning and operating your own streamlined fitness business, with reliable employees, predictable, consistent income, and the freedom to make your own schedule! I want to make that dream a reality for you. **Fitness Launch Formula** is my life's work, providing the complete framework needed to take your passion for fitness and transform it into a profitable career doing what you love.

Here are four agreements you need to make with yourself before we continue. Belief is everything. You will never be bigger than your own self concept, so before we begin, I ask that you speak these four agreements out loud and really let them settle into the deepest part of your being.

1 I believe I have a special gift that the world needs, and I have a strong desire to package that gift into products, programs and services that consumers will buy.

2 I believe in hard work, and I am someone who does not quit when I encounter an obstacle. I will always find a way to transcend my adversity. There is no "Plan B."

3 I believe in myself, my abilities, and my natural talents. They will take me to places I never thought possible.

4 I believe that I can do this! I know deep down I was created for something bigger than my current circumstances and I am ready to take the leap.

The World is Changing

Not long ago, making a living in the fitness industry meant working for a big-box gym, sports team, or university. There were no personal training studios with independent contractors, or niche brands that capitalized on a certain style of exercise, environment, or culture.

Then, one by one, fitness pros started to break the mold, and training facilities started popping up all over the place. Some did well and some crashed and burned, but one thing is for certain: the world of fitness had changed.

Today the options are endless. With the use of video, social media and blogging, fitness enthusiasts have been able to forge amazing careers out of simple ideas like hand balancing, windmill pitching, shoulder strengthening, fat loss camps, parkour, street dancing and more.

Now, by having a passion in the field of fitness and knowing 20% more about it than the next person, you have a viable business idea. The only thing you need is a platform, content, programs and a tribe. You can hold a master's degree in kinesiology or be a high-school dropout and the new rules of fitness business success apply equally to you as long as you follow the path I have outlined in this book.

Unfortunately for some, today's fitness industry has leveled the playing field. A degree, multiple certifications, and networking prowess don't necessarily guarantee success, nor does hefty financial backing. In the end, the success stories come from people who didn't give up, and set the stage for predictable customer satisfaction, streamlined back-end operations, calculated marketing, and scalability through very deliberate systems.

Isn't it comforting to know that you don't have to be an expert to earn a handsome income? In fact, you don't need much of anything to get started, except for one very important thing. You must have an intense, driving force propelling you forward, launching you into the fitness arena with reckless abandon. Many of those who possess this sort of passion start as "nobodies," but in just a few short years they've made their millions, continue to thrive while having more and more free time, and consistently retain loyal, massive tribes.

Perhaps my story will resonate (and if it doesn't, you're probably ahead of the curve!). I remember witnessing my father's disappointment as he held the phone to his ear. It was my high school principal, and he wasn't happy: "Brian will be lucky if he ends up driving a forklift. My bet is that he will be in jail within five years with this kind of behavior."

My principal was right. I had a knack for getting into trouble, disrupting class, and skipping out when something more interesting came along. I flunked out during my first year at Penn State, and was luckily (and generously) allowed back under a provisional status. I did manage to graduate six years later with dozens of extra credits though.

To showcase my defiance, upon graduation, instead of entering the workforce, I signed up for the Coast Guard and began a journey wrought with hard lessons and self-discovery. It became quite obvious that I was built a little differently than those around me (how could I not be, with that rap sheet!). It also became obvious that underneath some bad habits, bad history, and strained relationships, I had a very palpable, very influential passion. That passion was fitness.

When you know what you love, and that love is something that can be monetized, you start looking at the world differently. Those "nobodies" all had a moment when they realized the world was not there to put them down or stand in their way. It was and is an endless highway of opportunity. They changed their mindset, they changed their approach and they modeled what was working. So did I.

This mindset helped me to open six different brick-and-mortar health and fitness facilities without a hitch. During the process I derived a repeatable system that models the framework of a successful start-up process, which will be shared with you in this book.

I am confident that by sticking to the program and setting specific protocols in place now, you will have avoided the financially-draining and energy-depleting activities that end up drowning otherwise promising fitness businesses.

This system will help you effectively blueprint, brand, validate and test your ideas without spending a ton of money. You will know beyond a shadow of a doubt if your idea will make money before you even look for a site location, sign a lease, or apply for a loan.

The method is called **Fitness Launch Formula** and it has generated more than 3 million dollars in revenue across two simple brands. I have held this information close to my chest for years, allowing access to high-level private coaching clients only.

But in looking back to my earlier years, I realized what this information could have done for me. I believe that my career would have seen exponential return, and so I share it all with you in excitement for your venture into the not-so-scary unknown.

Now, if you're one of those "prove it" folks like me, you're probably wondering if I walk the walk. Here's what I've got: This book is a compilation of knowledge gained from 15 years in business and over $3 million in sales since 2008. It is the very simple, very repeatable method that has been tweaked, honed, and crafted through failures, triumphs, and many sleepless nights. Now all you have to do is read!

The Big Blue Mat

I've been where you may be right now. I've felt the pain of working endless hours and holidays for people I didn't respect or trust. I've been treated like a towel boy and spent years getting up at 4 a.m., only to return home at 7 p.m., too exhausted to make dinner, shower, or walk to the mailbox.

I worked for years only to lose everything when a greedy gym owner decided he wanted more of my income. I've struggled beyond what any person should, and I am here to tell you today that there is a better way.

Not long ago I was standing on the "big blue mat" at a training studio, where I worked as an independent contractor. There I was, counting reps and wondering if my life would ever change.

Though I loved fitness, I was standing for hours, counting reps, and hating my life.

I'd recently broken up with my fiance, which had sent me into a depressive tailspin. Still, my job required punctuality, creativity, and a plastered smile on my face hour after hour. Though painful, I could manage these criteria. What I couldn't manage was the most important job requirement: motivating others. How could I possibly create excitement and enthusiasm in someone else if I was dying inside?

And then of course, were the more pervasive, incessant questions looming from the break-up: Will I ever own my own gym, be an industry leader, get married or have a family? I wondered if I would ever matter beyond my ability to count and smile.

One day while standing on that big blue mat, a client made it a point to tell me that my programming style was so unique and effective compared to what he had experienced anywhere before.

As the day progressed, a few more clients shared the same sentiment. After sharing this news with a client who also happened to be a wealthy businessman, he encouraged me to start recording my workouts so as to reach a larger audience, and, of course, benefit financially from that larger audience.

So immediately I went to work. Research led me to a relatively unknown video hosting site, designed for personal video postings, and touted as a place to "get noticed." It was called YouTube. I say this in jest because at the time it was not the mega platform it is today. So I made a few videos with one of my friends, who traded her modeling time for free training. One night after work, I posted them to YouTube, scarfed down some food, and passed out.

The next morning, I knew my life had changed. The two training videos we haphazardly pieced together had gone viral overnight. As I brewed coffee and sat down to check my email, my jaw dropped. In a matter of hours I had been bombarded with messages from trainers around the world who were grateful for new material and hungry for more. They wanted to get inside my head and understand how to produce dynamic, efficient, and results-driven metabolic sequences like those shown in my videos.

I scrolled through my emails until my coffee was cold, and found myself driving to work in a dumbfounded stupor, mesmerized by the possibilities.

There was still a piece of me that doubted the legitimacy of those emails, and doubted the sincerity of the compliments regarding my programming. Did they know that it was the same college-floundering, fiance-losing, prison-bound Brian Devlin that produced those videos?

Despite a suspicious feeling that the joke might be on me, I reluctantly put a basic website together and continued posting more videos to YouTube, with links back to my site.

A client who had used email marketing to grow a charity, told me to join Constant Contact's newsletter service, and in doing so, they provided an email-capture to be used on my website. So my little template website now had a "subscribe for weekly videos" email-capture.

Within a month's time, I had accumulated more than 2,000 subscribers, all from YouTube traffic. So I did a little more research and purchased an online program to help me design a list building, email newsletter, which I then mailed to my subscribers weekly and asked them to share with their friends. The content was this: An inspirational pep talk (the break-up had primed me for some seriously powerful material), and two brief exercise videos outlining workouts that could be done with personal training clients. My newsletter went viral.

My subscribers loved the videos, and within months, asked me to release a training DVD, so that's exactly what I did. This was shot on a $300 camera and edited using Windows Movie Maker. The whole DVD took me three hours to shoot and edit from start to finish, and I burned it on my laptop. The title was "Core Salvation," and I informed my email list that the DVD would be on sale as soon as I could "figure out a way to sell stuff online " - no joke.

I went back to work, and this time I was more focused. I held a deeper belief in myself and was now determined to make this next business happen. I went to a couple of internet marketing forums and started asking questions.

As I was uploading videos one night, I stumbled on a blog about moonlighting on the internet. The site was run by a guy named Yanik Silver, and he was selling a program called "Yanik's Brain In A Box," with a whopping price tag of $2,000. His only disclaimer was: "If, after applying my information, you do not make this much money in eight weeks, I will personally help you or give you a full refund!"

My Insane Leap of Faith

I did it. I took the leap and went all in. The product arrived in a huge box about two weeks later and it was packed with what seemed like 50 DVDs and 20 manuals. Though already tight for time, I made a commitment to follow the steps necessary to set up my online shopping cart and blog using outsourced labor from India, per Yanik's advice.

The course taught me how to make a sales page and integrate the sales page with a shopping cart software program. The shopping cart software would take a payment and send automatic emails to a fulfilment company where my master DVD was stored. The fulfillment company would then ship the DVD to the appropriate address, anywhere in the world.

I had created a system that ran without me, start to finish, and it was the most liberating feeling in the world. Aside from the up-front work involved in creating the DVD, which I only had to do once, I expended no more energy beyond checking my bank account.

My First Taste of Automated Income

Well, once I tested the system with my own credit card and had my friend test it as well, I sent an email to my list and officially launched my DVD. The sales came in almost immediately. My bank account grew while I ate, while I read, while I worked, and the sweetest of all pleasures: it grew while I slept. I started going to work with a smile plastered on my face, but this time it was for good reason. In five days I had generated $5,000. I was on my way to freeing myself from the grind of personal training 10 hours a day.

The same trend continued for about two weeks and then sales started to screech to a halt. That experience will sober you up in no time. I emailed out but nobody else wanted to buy my DVD. I didn't understand; of the 3,000 subscribers only 150 had purchased the DVD. What had I done wrong?

My imagination had gotten the best of me, and my dreams of retiring in a year screeched to an abrupt halt. I immediately took interest in buying trends, only to find that what had happened was normal. In fact, at any given time, only about 10%-20% of your market will actually buy what you are selling. So the key is to constantly increase the size of your list or your market.

This was the first step I took toward developing the method that you are going to learn in this book. I had no idea it was going to become a piece of the launch formula at the time. I thought I had just learned my limitations.

I will dive more into this story later in the book because there are some key points that have emerged from this trial-and-error period. After I launched my online business, I used the income generated to bankroll my first fitness facility. I used the lessons from blogging and internet selling to create automation around generating leads and customer communication -- assets which quickly set me apart from others in the fitness industry.

Since 2008, my companies have generated more than $3 million in fitness-related revenue. I have opened four successful fitness locations and co-opened two successful chiropractic offices. My online coaching programs reached members in 48 states and 23 countries, and

I have personally coached dozens of struggling and successful fitness pros to use the methods I will discuss in this book.

Some of my students have gone on to open successful six- and seven-figure fitness ventures by following this simple blueprint, and now you can take the reigns of your business with confidence. Know that you are already on your way to extraordinary success; you have this compass to guide you through the rough terrain and warn you when danger lies ahead. What do you have to lose?

Not Just For Me

This is not a book about internet marketing, but I thought I would give you a snapshot of my humbling entrepreneurial beginnings. With a backpack and $200 to my name, I started my training business in Charleston, South Carolina. I drove a 1991 Mazda B2200 pickup truck with faulty brakes and no air conditioning.

I did not take out a loan for my first facility; I built it piece by piece. Month after month I would take my profits and pay my rent, my bills, and spend the rest on food and new equipment. I literally built it from scratch. I scoured Craigslist for people who were throwing out fitness equipment. Their garbage was my gateway to business heaven. I never paid full price for anything. Goodwill and TJ Maxx provided my wardrobe, tuna and pasta provided my sustenance – every financial decision weighed in favor of business growth over personal luxuries and entertainment.

You may have more leniencies than I had at the time. What I can guarantee is that this formula will take you from novice to fitness facility connoisseur without having to sell a limb in the process. As long as you are motivated, the formula will help you open your boot camp, training studio, big-box gym, crossfit affiliate, or mobile training business. It doesn't matter. These concepts are universal to location, fitness genre, and owner profile. They will work across the entire services industry.

You don't even have to rent a commercial facility. You can apply this model to a park or your own garage and work up from there. "Rome wasn't built in a day." You may not be in position to get a loan and that's OK! There is always a way; when you have a formula, you can start small and know exactly where you need to go once you gain momentum.

I challenge you to finish this book, get out there, and make your dream a reality. The chances of failure are practically non-existent as long as you adhere to the four agreements we discussed.

Why am I able to make such a bold claim? Track record. I have tested this system across multiple industries and multiple offerings. I have used it to help newbies and pros alike. Now, you will still make some mistakes. That's just life. Business perfection is an oxymoron. The only mistakes that matter are the ones that aren't addressed. With this formula, you'll be able to get started, quickly see where you need work, and make improvements until you're living and breathing your own dream.

Let's set a course together and nail this business thing once and for all!

CHAPTER ONE

The New Fitness Industry

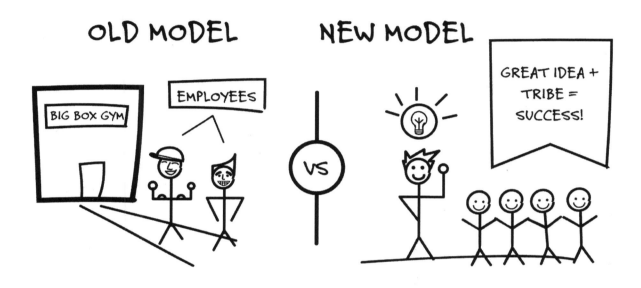

The Good

As stated in the introduction, we are in a new fitness industry and it's changing by the minute. Crossfit has brought functional metabolic fitness to the forefront of consumer awareness. People are interested in lifting weights as much as they want community and challenge. They want recognition and direction. They want a path that can take them to levels of function they have never imagined.

Your potential for creating an offering the public will accept has never been better. The Tough Mudder, Crossfit, X-games and extreme sports have paved hundreds of new avenues to sell fitness products, programs and services to your market. Things have changed in such a dramatic and exciting manner that by branding and creating a customer path around any fitness activity, you can not only create a viable business model, but a killer brand as well.

Look at Pure Barre. They have created a killer cult following centered on ballet workouts. Look at pole dancing. What used to be reserved for strippers and strip clubs is now available to moms who want to learn how to perform pole fitness. Look at aerial silks. What was once only seen in high-end Las Vegas shows is now being taught in every major city.

I could go on listing dozens and dozens of obscure fitness offerings that are absolute killer brands, but you get the point: Opportunity is endless! You have the world at your fingertips and the next million-dollar fitness business is right around the corner. When you put the **Fitness Launch Formula** framework to use, you can create multiple six- and seven-figure brands.

Are you pumped yet? If not, you should be. There has never been a better time to be in the fitness business. With YouTube, Wordpress, Facebook, software and apps, building a killer platform to test your ideas has never been easier.

The days of hope marketing are over. Now you can strategically place yourself directly in front of your target audience and validate your market before you spend a dime on a business venture.

The Bad

Even with the advances in technology and detailed blueprints out there, most trainers and fitness professionals are just too overwhelmed to take action and learn how to use these tools to test ideas and produce income. The average trainer in the United States makes less than 27K a year.

They still go to work every day wondering if they will ever be able to branch off and claim their own facility, fill it with employees, and generate a healthy dependable income to feed a family.

They stand there counting reps and struggle to stay awake because they have been up since 4 a.m. and they still have five evening clients to meet across town. They are doing everything wrong, yet still get results for their clients.

Clients love their trainers, and trainers hate their clients for stealing the time and the energy it would take to get motivated at the end of the day. So the trainers resentfully stand and count, and do it all again tomorrow. The only thing they look forward to is putting their headphones on, taking their pre-workout drink, and busting out their own stress-relieving workout.

I know this because I interview a lot of frustrated trainers during the free strategy calls I offer from time to time. They all start off by saying they think they need help getting more clients and learning to market, and they end the call realizing they need to love what they are doing and build scalability into their life. This is what I do. I am an automation engineer. I am a delegation master. I don't do anything I don't want to do, and this is how you have to be if you want to launch a killer brand.

The Ugly

Most trainers will read this book, get super-excited, start phase one of the formula and then quit before they validate their idea. How do I know this? Because for years I had the number one coaching program for personal trainers called The Underground Fitness Formula. It was a monster. There were three parts to it: High-performance business, high-performance programming and high-performance marketing. Every month my team of successful facility owners would share what was working "now" in those three categories, and we would provide three types of homework. Each member had a video lesson and then homework in the three key areas.

We had more than 250 members paying $47 a month to have access to the information and the community. Of the 250 members, about 20 opened successful facilities during that coaching program. The other 230 did very little after the first week.

Why would someone spend $47 a month on a program that they never even used? The same reason people spend $40 a month on a gym membership and go three times a year. They have no follow-through.

Are they bad people? No. Are they lazy? Probably not. They are just average. They are the 90%. If you want to be a business owner and you want to build a fitness business you love while living a life of freedom, you have to dedicate yourself to being the 10%. Only 10% of people who set out to open a business will ever get it off the ground. The only thing that is keeping them from doing it is their own belief system.

You have got to believe that you were created for something great. You were designed with talents, skills and a true purpose. The world needs what you have inside of you and you have to be dedicated to nurturing that gift. That purpose will expand with reckless abandon as soon as you recognize that it exists and start making decisions with that in mind.

Until you change your mindset, this book and any other educational course will still leave you in the realm of the 90%. Believe you are the 10%. Rise above your excuses. Rise above saying, "You don't understand, Brian. My situation is different." Sure it may be different, but it is not unique in the world. Somewhere, somebody with a crappy hand is playing cards like a boss. Don't be the 90% complaining about the odds.

If you want to make it in this business you gotta play your cards like a boss, and I'm about to show you how that is done.

The **Fitness Launch Formula** is an eight-phase process that takes you from the foundational elements of your business identity to your grand opening.

I will label the phases, then tell you a little more about myself and the mistakes I have made while putting this framework together. So don't read ahead because I don't want you to miss the application nuggets that I have buried in my personal story.

Without these application points, you will have a much harder time understanding the **Fitness Launch Formula** in its entirety.

These eight phases are made up of action steps you will need to complete in order to move into the next phase. Each action is chronologically ordered so that you can easily work from Phase 1 to Phase 8. The book is laid out so you can complete one action step per day, but you are welcome to do more than one if you desire.

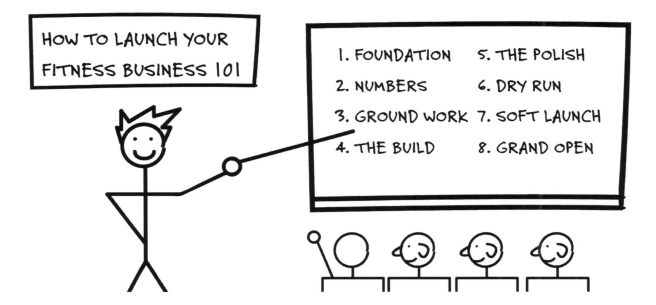

HOW TO LAUNCH YOUR FITNESS BUSINESS 101

1. FOUNDATION   5. THE POLISH

2. NUMBERS   6. DRY RUN

3. GROUND WORK   7. SOFT LAUNCH

4. THE BUILD   8. GRAND OPEN

The First Phase is the foundational work. This is where you work through the process of building a killer brand. This can take up to 11 days and will require a lot of personal quiet time so you can get down to the heart of the matter at hand.

The Second Phase will talk about numbers, projections and metrics. This is where you work through your processes, validate your business model and determine if your offering is viable enough to seek financing or invest your money.

The Third Phase is the groundwork phase. This is a hard phase and usually separates the 90% from the 10%. If you make it through this phase, your chances of success go way up and you should consider yourself a business owner.

The Fourth Phase is the build-out phase. This is when you get your hands dirty and become fully committed to your venture financially and emotionally. During this phase, your facility will take shape and you will know what you need to do in every step of the way to get it opened and running smoothly.

The Fifth Phase is the polishing phase. It's when you tie up loose ends, obtain your certificate of occupancy, wrap up the detail work and get ready to start testing your systems thoroughly.

The Sixth Phase is the dry-run training phase. During this phase, you use test subjects to work through the entire customer process, then complete your facility audit. You get feedback needed to make the necessary changes and prepare for your soft launch.

The Seventh Phase is the soft launch phase. This is where you draw a select number of targeted leads into your funnel and run them through, just like you would for a grand opening. You gather final feedback, make the needed adjustments to your systems and your facility and prepare for your grand opening.

The Final Phase is where you plan and execute your grand opening and go through your proprietary post-opening activities that we will cover in detail. After this, your business is officially launched and can now enter the second realm, which we will cover in my next book. We will touch on some post-opening steps in this book that you can take that will ensure the growth and prosperity of your new venture.

You may be wondering how I stumbled on this unique method of opening a fitness business, and the answer is not very exciting. Every key point I cover in this launch sequence is something I screwed up in the past, or something my coaching clients screwed up when they launched their business. I have distilled all my mistakes and all my successes into a simple action plan that you can follow to the letter and hopefully achieve the same level of success I have had — or better. I remember posting in a Facebook group that I was fortunate enough to break the $3 million mark in personal training sales with my facilities and offered some advice on how to get unstuck. The response was positive, but disbelieving. Most people could not believe that I had generated so many sales in a niche that is often referred to as "dead."

No niche is dead. Only the methods you use to market to that niche die. This is the new fitness industry and I am here to show you how to make your passion profitable for years to come. Before we dive into the eight-fold framework for launching your business the right way, let's back up. I want to give you a little look into where my passion began. Your story is likely far different from mine, but it is important to rediscover where **your** passion began. There will be moments when you will need a reminder of this story to propel you forward. It will ignite your journey when the going gets tough, and will constantly redirect you to your place in the 10%.

CHAPTER TWO

A Crash Course In My Personal Theology

Theology: The supporting rationale, doctrine, beliefs, tenets and written word that backs up and confirms what the voice in your head is telling you.

The Urban Dictionary

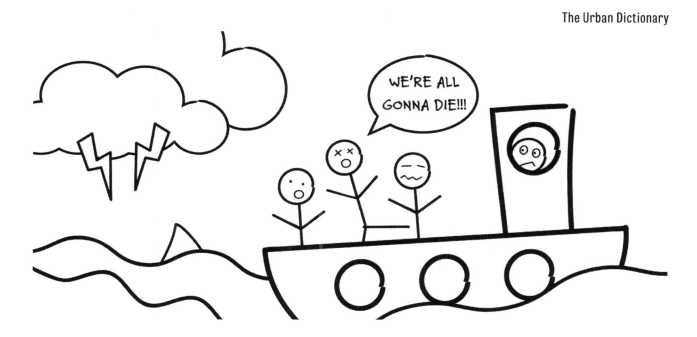

"**Brian! I** want to see my wife and kids again. Please get us home." I will never forget those words. They still haunt me to this day. They were so short, intense and powerful that I still get goose bumps thinking about them.

Petty Officer Sarver was my crew engineer that day. He was in charge of making sure the engines never stopped running and the water never entered the cabin. My job was to ensure that we came home alive. I was the captain of the Coast Guard 41-foot rescue boat and it was my job to make sure we completed the mission without incident.

It was nightfall in Dauphin Island, Alabama, situated at the mouth of Mobile Bay on the shores of the Gulf of Mexico. We had just received a call from a fishing boat seven miles offshore with a crew-member emergency. One of the fishing crew had apparently suffered a heart attack and could not maintain consciousness.

We had received the latitude and longitude from our command in Mobile and were proceeding south, down the Mobile ship channel at 25 knots. It was dark and radar showed a slew of incoming freighters in the channel.

The wind was blowing hard and the last four miles of the channel looked like a washing machine from hell. All I could see was spray, a crappy radar image of our incoming freighter traffic, and huge, confused breaking surf.

The safe operating limitations of a Coast Guard UTB are six-foot seas and 30-knot winds. I am here to tell you that conditions in the channel exceeded the operational limitations of my rescue craft. My crew and I were in danger. As we narrowly passed the 700-foot freighters and were tossed by their bow shear, I remember looking out at the sea in front of me. I was looking for my landmark. I needed to find my range marker.

A range marker is a series of two lights with different flashing intervals. If you are in the channel, the faster flash will appear directly below the slower flash. You know you are left or right of the channel when these distant lights appear to deviate. I could not see my range markers anymore. I asked my crewman to find the ranges on the radar, but he was unable to pull them up.

We were headed into a huge squall and things were about to get rough. I remember when the first wave hit. It rose up in front of us like a towering giant and drove fear into my heart. My first reaction was to accelerate and power up the beast, but it was too late. It broke right on the cabin and completely engulfed us with a wall of water.

I yelled at everyone to hold on as a second wave hit us dead on the bow. This time the wall hit us like a sledgehammer. It smashed on the windshield and made a sound that still raises the hair on my head, like the cross between a knockout punch and an open-hand slap from God himself. The boat shuttered and creaked. My crew was mute. It was then that Sarver broke the silence and said those words I will never forget.

Just then, we were hit on the beam by a crashing wave and the boat listed hard to port about 35 degrees and then back to starboard. McCormick went flying into the bulkhead on the other side of the cabin and McCloskey soon followed.

At this point I was actually scared. The 41-foot UTB has been known to capsize, and every time it had capsized it resulted in loss of life. We were in a real situation and it was up to me to get us out. I remember thinking to myself, "I am not ready to die." I was afraid and I started to ask myself and God a whole bunch of serious questions.

Like the storm itself, the flood of questions began: "Why the hell am I here? What am I doing in this town? Why am I doing this work?" I didn't even want to drive boats. I joined the Coast Guard to be a helicopter rescue man. The school was full when I graduated boot camp, so I opted to be a boat captain instead, because it was the only way I would see land. The aviation program had a three-year waiting list, which my friendly recruiter failed to divulge at the time of enlistment. Go figure.

I replayed my life in my head. I remembered moments with my siblings as a child, getting my heart broken in college, my parents and how poorly we left things as I drove off to Alabama without looking back. I felt a deep sadness overcome my whole body, realizing we may capsize and I would never have really lived. I would have left my family with unresolved pain; I would never have known what it felt like to have the love of a wife, or experienced the day my child called me Daddy.

Then I started to think about my crew and their hopes and dreams. I thought about Sarver's wife and McCormick's kids as they found out their husbands and fathers were lost at sea. I asked God if it was our time. I never heard his voice but I did receive a message. "You have not used your gift yet."

I sat there for a moment and contemplated this burst of revelation. I didn't even know I had a gift. I never even looked at life through those eyes. I was just concerned about the next experience or the next distraction.

I remember this feeling of amazing calm engulfing my body. I looked around at my crew and could see the terror in their eyes. I looked at the ocean in front of me and it seemed to be taunting me. But I was somehow removed from it, protected from it. The waves were crashing into the cabin and the movie played in slow motion. I watched as the bull-nose crashed below the surface. The water shot at us like a cannon in slow motion; the boat engines whined as if the ocean itself had a hold on the propeller shafts.

I took the throttles in my hands and the wheel jerked back and forth with the surges of the beam seas. I fixed my eyes on the Mobile Sea Buoy, which was about a mile off my bow. It was violently swaying from side to side but I knew that was our safe zone. We would be south of the breaking bar and out of real danger from capsizing in minutes. The washing machine that had threatened us no longer held me captive with fear.

Somehow deep down in my spirit I knew that God himself spoke to me and ushered in a new era, the era of self-awareness. No longer would I live for the moment or the next exciting outing. From this day forward, I would search deep within until I found my gift. I knew this gift would lead me to do great and mighty things. It would lead me to inspire thousands. I heard it in my spirit and I couldn't ignore its command. The command clearly stated: "Your gift will make room for you and bring you before great and mighty men."

The purpose of this book is to help you find your true gift and launch it into a lasting career that will bring you income and fulfillment for years to come. I want you to uncover your real power plant. This awareness and revelation will remove the guesswork from the rest of your life. It will give you a clear and detailed blueprint for why you are here and where you should be focusing your greatest efforts. You have been issued a weapon. This weapon is your gift and it will help you overcome many adversaries.

It will carve out phenomenon and wonder in your everyday existence, if you let it. You have to see life as a true journey and a genuine adventure in order to really understand and become a practitioner of your own theology.

I am not here to tell you how or who to worship. I am not here to sell you a religion or lead you to salvation. I am here to pull back the curtain and help you find your real power plant. I'm here to help you see yourself, your life and your purpose with a completely different set of eyes. I want you to have eyes that see. When you have eyes that see, ears that hear and a heart that is truly decided, your life will take on new meaning and new wonder. You won't see all the legwork that lies ahead in the following chapters as painful tasks you must force yourself to complete. You will see the required work list as GPS way points on your chosen path of desire, meaning and service.

I promise by the time you finish reading this guide, your personal theology will be deeply ingrained into your psyche, your heart and your soul. You will know your dream and the steps required to bring it to fruition. You will have a power plant that does not have blackouts, does not lose energy and forever powers your passion.

You will have a desire to go deeper than you have ever gone. Deeper into yourself. Deeper into your relationships, and deeper into serving others. You will navigate sticking points and pitfalls because you have a decided heart. Once a man decides in his heart he desires a thing, not even the devil himself can derail his dream. When you become clear, your world becomes clear. You attract like-minded people and you form strong unions. You have a gift. It will take you on an amazing adventure of tenacity, triumph and tears. I am your guide. I will do my best to instill my 30,000 hours of real life experience into your journey.

Let it begin as we look at your way points on this path to success.

I have used the process set out in the following chapters to do almost everything in my life. It is a blueprint for success online and offline. I have used this blueprint with private coaching clients and with my own businesses online and offline. It works! Plain and simple. This is the sole reason I have been able to live a lifestyle I designed from scratch from my own theology, and break the $3 million mark selling something I truly believe in. I want to pass this knowledge on to you and I only ask that you use the information in the following pages to help people and serve others. When you do this, you will never want or need anything.

CHAPTER THREE

The Tested Launch Formula

Let's dive in. What makes the **Fitness Launch Formula** so successful? This is a question I get asked a lot, and here's my best answer:

The success comes from the way your activities are stacked and the order in which you execute the action plan. Completing these steps haphazardly will really throw off the effectiveness of the formula, and your energy will be poorly spent sorting through hiccups and bottlenecks that could have otherwise been avoided. The **Fitness Launch Formula** framework is explained in explicit detail later in the book, but this chapter will help you understand why you can easily implement this formula into any fitness offering with unparalleled success.

In Phase 1 of the formula, we go through the right actions to ensure your brand and business model are rock solid: You have a long-term vision, you know what you want to accomplish, you have an idea of what your end game will be, and you have actually validated (not just selected) your niche market.

This is so important to do first. Because if you don't have an architecture for your business idea and you are just going on hunches, you are engaging in a suicidal business venture that will continue to become an uphill battle for you and your team in the future. Know your end game before you make your first move. This is a skill that separates millionaires from has-beens.

The number one reason most professional athletes are broke within a few years of retirement is that they fail to see their end game ahead of time. They are caught up in celebrity status and huge paychecks, but fail to develop a long-term brand that will generate income for them long after their fame fades.

Michael Jordan is a great example of someone who saw his end game while he was still a star athlete, and now owns many businesses that will take care of him for years to come.

In Phase 2, I will take you through some vital activities and calculations to first determine if you are heading in the right direction with your business idea. There is no sense investing in a business idea that the market will not embrace, or investing in a business that has no viable customers in your area. When you go through the exercises in Phase 2, you will quickly be able to tell if your idea is viable and if you have an actual market demographic that would invest in your idea.

You will also be moved through some vital exercises that help maximize your pricing models for top conversions and long-term profit. There is a sweet spot, and until you find that spot you may be leaving money on the table.

The Disney Corporation is a perfect example of a company that really spent some time researching its market and developing pricing for maximum effectiveness and long-term growth. The way they have their products, programs and services arranged helps them hit all facets of the market and enables them to offer low-, mid-, and high-tier programs to customers, always giving them a reason to ascend to the next level of investment.

In Phase 3, we move out of blueprinting and into actually getting your hands dirty. We cover activities needed to secure the right location, how to ask the right questions when it comes to lease negotiation, some pitfalls to look out for, and how to get through local codes and restrictions with a minimum financial investment.

When we have an idea that works and we know how to navigate the red tape surrounding the execution of that idea, we are able to increase our speed of implementation and time to market. This gives us a huge advantage over the competition, because we can implement a money-making strategy faster and take advantage of the initial free rent we may be receiving from effective lease negotiation strategies.

We are also able to acquire the necessary financing to get our venture off the ground when we know ahead of time what banks will require of us, and the common interest rates that private lenders and silent investors charge. This section will help you avoid the pitfalls of getting in bed with the wrong business partner and allow you to forecast the future liability and asset margin you will hold in your company as time progresses.

Don't let big financial words frighten you. I have been running businesses for 15 years and I have encountered many big words that, when explained, were actually very easy to understand and basically boiled down to common-sense math.

In Phase 4, we will start to have fun with our business because we finally get to build it. We can do the fun stuff like researching equipment, selecting flooring, finding contractors and getting our venture on the map and ready for our final tweaks and polish. During this phase, you will start to see all of your groundwork pay off. This is always where I start to get a little nervous, seeing the mountain of liabilities grow in front of me. Keep your story ever-present in your mind during this phase, and know that with great risk comes great reward.

By giving you a snapshot of what's to come, your fears should be dwindling. You have the power to charge ahead with gusto and take your business by the horns, facing all your fears head-on because you are following a model that has yielded millions in sales with unbeatable profit margins. As you progress and overcome hurdles along your destined path, your confidence will swell and the journey to the finish line will become a self-perpetuating ride to excitement and success.

This is where you get to be totally you. Customize and implement the information as you see fit, while still sticking to the general architecture of this formula. **Fitness Launch Formula** is like a franchise handbook without the fees and rules. You get to use a proven system while maintaining the freedom to do it with your own unique offering.

In Phase 5, we will take out our microscope and polish your business so that you are ready to impress your test-clients and turn them into raving fans. This is the type of preparation and polish that very few business owners apply. It is the secret sauce that has allowed me to open six facilities in different niches without a hitch or a complaint. We will address activities you need to undertake to ensure that your test subjects not only love your offering, but are literally telling everyone they know about your business before you even open. Going into your soft launch, you will most likely profit, and it will all be due to some simple actions you took that nobody else did.

In Phase 6 of your launch, you will complete your dry-run training, find test clients and make them an offer they absolutely cannot refuse. You will gather data, take pictures, survey and more. Then we will take all this data and use it to become the best offering within miles of your new facility; the interest will be so great, people will be throwing money at you in anticipation of your soft launch. We will do this through a special form of re-targeting. The results may be nothing short of miraculous. I feel confident in saying that if you follow the steps in this phase your chances of failing will be nearly zero.

In Phase 7, you will have your soft opening and we will bring our tweaked and polished program to a set number of users and really test the limitations, if any, of our model. The activities we will cover in this phase will bring us to our grand opening with little effort. By this time, we will have ironed out 90% of the kinks, and will be focusing on that last 10% before we launch our business to the public on a large scale. Depending on the scope of our business and the size of our facility, a soft launch may be the end of the road for our launch formula. I have opened, and helped to open, many businesses that never really had a grand opening. But we will cover your grand opening procedure in detail in the eighth and final phase in case you choose to have one.

At that point in the launch formula, we take your gift, which is all wrapped up and packaged into a finely tuned, integrated product suite, and we deliver it to the world in a big way. We have a grand opening event and we get massive exposure to really put you on the map as far as a business goes. The activities we will cover in this chapter are completely optional and you may or may not want to invest in a grand opening event. They do cost money and they don't always increase your bottom line, but in many cases they are very effective in convincing prospects of your credibility, especially if you have a speaker and media coverage.

The phases in my launch formula are broken down into chapters, and each phase is divided into activities to complete each day. There is one activity per day because I don't want you to feel overwhelmed. But you are more than welcome to complete more than one activity each day depending on the amount of time you have to commit to the prescribed tasks.

At the end of each chapter you will see some resources that can be used to expand your understanding of certain concepts I touch on, highlight a special tool I use, or offer a deeper level of training you may be interested in pursuing to streamline the growth and automation of your business after launch.

CHAPTER FOUR

Business Foundation & Identity

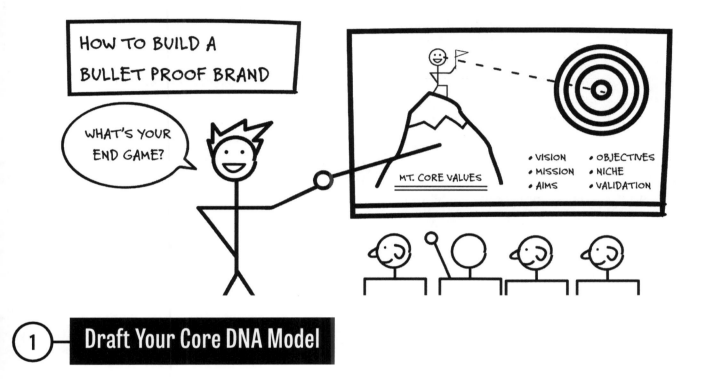

1 — Draft Your Core DNA Model

Our core DNA is the skeletal structure that makes up our company's core identity and it is far more important than you might think. But before you can construct your core identity, you must first ask yourself these three very hard questions.

Who Am I?

Who are you at the deepest level? What are you? What is your concept of self? What do you see when you look in the mirror, see yourself in pictures, or listen to the sound of your own voice? Do you like it? Do you wish it were different? What would you change? What are you lying about? These are some extremely personal, emotional and hard questions I have had to ask myself, and you should too. They will unlock your true nature and what you can really expect from yourself and your business.

What we believe ourselves to be is vital to long-term vision, mission aims and objectives that we will need when we construct our Corporate DNA later on.

Why Am I Here And What Is My True Purpose?

Why are you alive? Are you here because of a random sperm and egg encounter years ago, or are you here because the world needs you? Did God bring you into being because there was a plan for your life, or are you just a random act of the ever-expanding universe?

When you come to the truth about who you are and what purpose you serve, you will have a hard time failing because your "why" will trump your circumstances. Let me be brutally honest. You will have many struggles getting your business from infancy to maturity, but if your "why" is stronger than your struggles you will always prevail. You will always dig deep and know that this is your destiny. It is what you were created to do. The cool thing about knowing your why is that your why will evolve. It will ebb and flow within you and it will take you down the path of life.

In some capacity, you will always know deep within your soul whether you are on or off your path. In my opinion, you can only be in one of two places, and if you listen you will always be able to return to the right place, the place that will bring your business and your life into alignment and inherently into great success.

What Do I Really Want And Why?

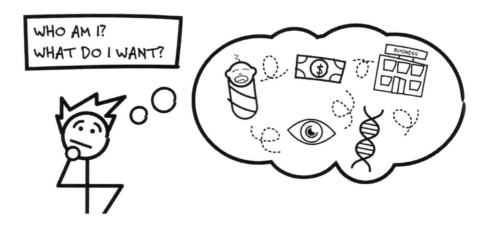

This is probably the one most people skim over; they do not dig deep into themselves and really explore what makes them happy, while ignoring the judgments they've heard in the past or placing judgment on themselves based on what they think is acceptable. They just react to their physiological state when presented with an idea. I have fallen victim to this many times. What you really want and what you think you want are usually very different. You may say I want a million dollars a year and to be able to travel the globe and party like a rock star. When this materializes, however, you could still find yourself extremely lonely and unfulfilled because you failed to combine it with the second part of the question.

If you ask why you want a million dollars and to travel the globe you may find that you really just don't want to worry about finances, and you want a life of new experiences and adventure. Well you don't have to make a million dollars and travel the globe to have what you really want, do you? Heck, you could do that with just a few hundred thousand and many impromptu trips and explorations in your local environment.

I wanted to own houses in a few areas of the U.S. so I could travel back and forth, and I wanted to make a passive 100K income that came in on autopilot, because I thought it would make me happy. I was so wrong. Owning multiple houses was stressful and even the idea of automated income came with its own set of worries. What would I do if and when my customers got bored or burned out and quit my programs? Would I be willing to trade time for money again to make the income necessary to sustain multiple homes? I certainly wouldn't be able to enjoy them with that work schedule.

When I decided to re-evaluate my life after the birth of my daughter, I realized that I didn't really want to travel all over, and having the extra income was nice but did not make me happy. So I sold my extra property and focused more on building a business in the town where I grew up so I could be closer to my aging family.

If I had realized long ago that I just wanted to be closer to those I love and have the financial freedom to make a move and start a new business, I would have done things much differently. I urge you to really dig deep and know the true answers to these three questions before continuing on.

Once you know deeply who you are, why you are here, and what you really want, proceed to the next phase.

(2) Define Your Core Values

This is crucial to long-term success because this will give you the ability to say "no" to all the wrong people, opportunities and things, and "yes" to all the right ones. Your core values make up your personal and professional compass, always guiding you in the direction of truth. They will ensure your decisions are congruent with your deepest beliefs. Stay true to your core values, because as soon as you act in opposition to your deepest beliefs, you will feel the backlash in your life and your business.

Download our "core values" worksheet to better understand your own core values, then place your top 5 core values in the spaces below before moving on.

Go here to download the core values worksheet: FitProEvolution.com/Core-Values/

Core Value 1 _____ Rating _____

Core Value 2 _____ Rating _____

Core Value 3 _____ Rating _____

Core Value 4 _____ Rating _____

Core Value 5 _____ Rating _____

Now that you have uncovered your real core values, work daily to bring those ratings up to a 10 in your day-to-day life. This will keep you on track and happy.

3 — Write Your Mission Statement

Your mission statement simply defines three things:

1 Your top business goals

2 Your best customer experience

3 How you provide that experience

It defines what your company stands for and who you are to your customers, employees, vendors, suppliers, and community. The best way to develop your own mission statement is to fill out the mission statement brainstorming worksheet, then look at the mission statements of successful companies and insert your own values, objectives and practices. Use vibrant words and make sure you are extremely satisfied with the end result.

Mission Checklist:

- Clear. simple and easily explained by others
- Not confused with a **vision** statement
- Recognizably your voice

? — What type of program/service do you offer?

_____

_____

? — What problems do you solve/needs do you meet?

_____

_____

? — What's the broadest way to describe your work?

_____

_____

? — For whom do you do this work?

_____

_____

? — Where do you work? (Geographical boundaries)

_____

_____

√ — Now write your Mission Statement:

_____

_____

Examples:

Livestrong: To inspire and empower people affected by cancer.

American Heart Association: To build healthier lives free of cardiovascular disease and stroke.

Harley-Davidson: We fulfill dreams through the experience of motorcycling, by providing to motorcyclists and the general public an expanding line of motorcycles and branded products and services in selected market segments.

Disney: To be one of the world's leading producers and providers of entertainment and information, using its portfolio of brands to differentiate its content, services and consumer products.

(4) Define Your Vision

Your vision statement is a vivid image of the future you wish to create for your business long term, and is not to be confused with your mission statement (who we are and what we do).

When I created my vision for Synergy Fitness, I saw it as a bicycle tire with the gym being at the center and all the spokes being my different points of leverage. I used the gym as a hub from which I created information products, software, coaching programs, membership sites and more. My vision for Synergy Fitness traveled way past the walls of the gym and covered the entire world.

My vision did not stop at providing services to patrons, but continued to trainers, gym owners and even business coaches.

Be bold when writing your vision statement because it outlines your biggest dream and grandest vision for your company.**The questions you must ask:**

? Why does your company exist?

_____

_____

? What will you be known for and where will it be known?

_____

_____

? Who is your target consumer or customer?

_____

_____

? — What are your company's financial goals?

_____

_____

? — What services will you provide for your customers?

_____

_____

? — Why will individuals want to become a member of your organization?

_____

_____

? — What is the culture of your organization?

_____

_____

? — What are the five keywords that sum up the scope of your vision:

1) _____

2) _____

3) _____

4) _____

5) _____

? — In three years what will your company look like?

_____

_____

? — In five years what will your company look like?

_____

_____

? — In 10 years what will your company look like?

_____

_____

√ — **Now compile your vision statement:**

_____

_____

(5) — Set the Aims and Objectives for Your Company

You should be feeling pretty good by now. You have done more than 75% of all fitness businesses operating world-wide have done already. The problem with most fitness professionals is that they have really big egos. Most fitness pros are too headstrong and too stubborn to actually admit they have no clue how to run a business or methodically run one. They tell themselves that their innate talent and skill will carry them through, and just like hitting PRs they will crush this business thing because they are disciplined.

You are right! You will crush it. You will be successful and desired and booked solid and you will also be miserable and here's why:

There is a certain thrill that comes with recognition. You will be recognized for your effort, your attitude, your results, and you will be placed on a pedestal. We are all human and the need for affirmation is deep within us. I love being affirmed and worshiped by my clients.

It's awesome, but it comes with a price. The price is freedom. You will be working 12-hour days and be unable to convince your clients to work with a new trainer, because you have groomed them to love, need and crave your expert guidance. You screwed up!

Let's face the facts. There are 16 waking hours in a day.

- 3 are spent eating?
- 6-8 are spent working?
- 2 are spent on personal time?

So you have 1-5 hours left to take care of everything else you need to run your business, make ends meet, schedule clients and take care of personal hygiene? Honestly, what kind of life is that?

That's not a life I am interested in, but it will be the life you lead unless you are willing to let go of ego, get your customer to fall in love with your systems and your employees and just respect you as the mastermind behind the big show.

In order to make this happen, you will need established aims and objectives for your customers and employees even if you have none right now. If you follow the framework I have laid out in this field guide, you won't have a problem attracting either.

What Are Your Aims?

Aims are specific outcomes you will bring about for your customers after they sign up for your fitness services. Anytime you are in a service-related industry there is an outcome or change that the client or customer is paying for.

? — What specific outcomes or change are you going to provide for your customer?

Specific Outcome 1: _____

_____

Specific Outcome 2: _____

_____

Specific Outcome 3: _____

_____

Specific Outcome 4: _____

_____

Specific Outcome 5: _____

_____

Specific Outcome 6: _____

_____

Specific Outcome 7: _____

_____

What Are Objectives?

Objectives are how you bring about change for your customers. What specific tactics and strategies are you going to use to ensure these changes are guaranteed?

? — What are the tools you have at your disposal and the tools you will employ to create these changes?

Tool or Strategy 1: _____

_____

Tool or Strategy 2: _____

_____

Tool or Strategy 3: _____

_____

Tool or Strategy 4: _____

_____

Tool or Strategy 4: _____

_____

Tool or Strategy 6: _____

_____

Tool or Strategy 7: _____

_____

Personal Promise:

I know these aims and objectives will set me apart from the pack. I know that they will require work to build and maintain, but I am committed to making this happen now so that in the very near future I can enjoy the fruits of strategic labor.

–Brian Devlin

Define Your War & Create Your Superhero Identity

Let's face it, we are at war. If we have nothing to oppose, nothing to eradicate, then we have no real reason to be in business. Think about this:

- A hair stylist who has a sloppy dye job and doesn't care about bad hair
- A scientist who is indifferent about accurate lab findings
- A chiropractor who does not care about providing pain relief

The above examples are people who have no real war or hatred for something they wish to eradicate. How do you think they will do in their business or career? Now look at these examples:

- A trainer who used to weigh 400 pounds and knows what it feels like to be overweight.
- A physical therapist who had a car accident and rehabbed major injuries back to 100%.
- A victim of physical abuse who became a therapist to help others

Which group will see more success? Which group will trigger massive change and become a hero to someone else?

I hope you chose the latter, because he who lacks passion and something to fight for will have no reason to stay the course. If your reason is money, you are already dead.

Nothing upsets me more than to see trainers talk about how they should be making six figures when they cannot show one case study of how they changed a life, or show one testimonial from a client who loved them for what they did.

Use the following worksheet to define your enemy and create the superhero within you, willing to seek out and eradicate the enemy.

Part 1: Niche Selection

What are my greatest strengths in fitness?

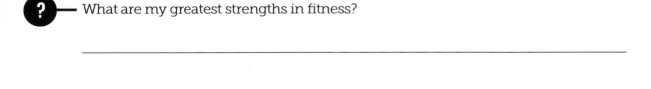

? — What can I teach better than anyone else?

_____

_____

? — What problem in fitness do I wish to eradicate permanently?

_____

_____

? — What do I love doing in fitness?

_____

_____

? — What do I hate doing in fitness?

_____

_____

? — Who do I love to work with in fitness? (Gender, age, problem)

_____

_____

? — Who do I hate to work with in fitness? (Gender, age, problem)

_____

_____

? — Do I like working in groups or privately? (Why?)

_____

_____

? — When do I like to work? (Morning, afternoon, evenings, weekends, all the time)

_____

_____

Now that you have identified your target market, take the market test below. If you get green lights you have a killer niche. If you don't get green lights, keep working because your target market is not adequate for a business venture.

Part 2: Niche Validation

To validate your niche, you need to know if the client you wish to attract is worth the time, money, and effort to rely on them for consistent income.

If you can answer five or more of the following questions with a "green light," you know you can count on your desired customer's loyalty; you can also feel confident about the style of gym you have chosen, the services you render, and to whom you're rendering them.

This is very important: Many of these questions are too broad for you to answer at this stage in the book, but I wanted to plant the seed now so that you can come back and validate your niche before taking real action steps toward site selection, etc.

The last thing you want to do is pursue a market that will not be fruitful, and the only way to do that is by completing the following list. After you have worked through the rest of **Fitness Launch Formula**, come back to this. Highlight it now. You can't move on without it.

Simply keep these questions in the back of your mind moving forward so that you can quickly and confidently answer them later.

? — Is your market big enough to max out your business model?

       Yes (Green Light)   No

? — Is the growth rate of your market active?

       Yes (Green Light)   No

? — Is there a lot of competition around your market?

       Yes   No (Green Light)

? — Are the current customers in your target market loyal to their current brand?

    Yes   No (Green Light)

? — Can you reach the majority of your target market easily through advertising?

    Yes (Green Light)   No

? — Is the sales potential for your target market adequate based on your pricing model?

    Yes (Green Light)   No

? — Is the expected profit margin of your market idea something that could max out your ideal projections?

    Yes (Green Light)   No

Add up your green lights and see below:

    5-7 Green Lights = Wide Open and Hot Niche - You Have A Winner

    3-4 Green Lights = Questionable Niche - Proceed With Caution

    0-3 Green Lights = Dead End Niche - Avoid At All Costs

Keep working with this until you really uncover a killer niche and then build your super-hero identity by learning how to solve every problem this niche has in a really cool and high-value way.

Big Takeaway

Always create high-value solutions to common problems your niche may be experiencing, and deliver those solutions through goodwill and generosity and you will never want for prospects, customers or employees.

CHAPTER FIVE

Metrics, Numbers And Demographics

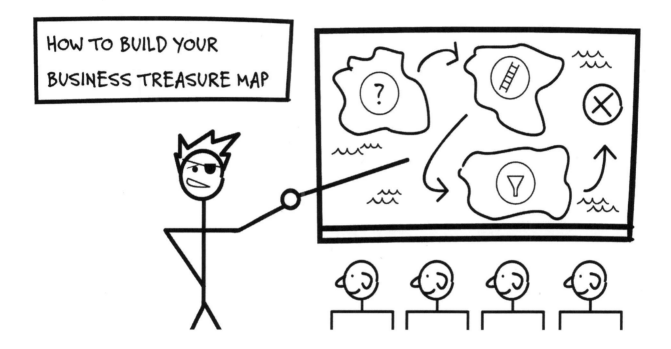

In this phase I will walk you step-by-step through the process of choosing your model, creating your program ladders, forecasting your numbers, setting your pricing, mapping out your conversion process and more!

This is probably the most tactical section of this book and I encourage you to devote enough time to thoroughly understand the concepts and strategies herein.

1 — Choosing Your Model

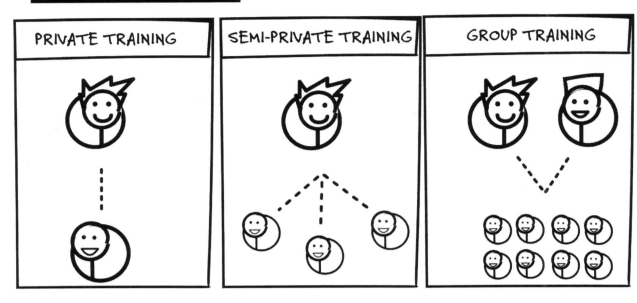

In terms of choosing your business model, there are generally three major models that work today, and there are endless variations on each of the three models. The first model is to have your business comprised of mainly private personal training clients. This is the model I use at my facility in Charleston, S.C., and it has worked amazingly well for me and my team.

I don't know you. I don't know your specific skills and talents, so the only advice I can offer to you is to choose wisely by validating your model selection using the same red light/green light method described in Chapter 4, Day 6.

The second model is semi-private training and it usually involves groups of 3-8 people. This type of training is usually a medium price point and has a medium level of attrition associated with it. The clients are trained in a circuit-based format and there is usually a high level of camaraderie within the group.

To use a semi-private model, you need enough space and enough equipment for your groups to function optimally. This can be pricey, so you may want to hold off on semi-private training until you have the capital.

The third and final model we will discuss is the group training model. In this model, one or two instructors train groups of 10-80 people in a room using mainly bodyweight training, mats, suspension trainers and dumbbells or kettle bells.

The programming is usually non-specialized and the clients don't expect much in terms of program supervision. Group training usually has a higher attrition rate than private and semi-private, and yields a much lower price-per-visit than the above models. The income is generated by sheer volume.

As you can see, all models above have their pros and cons and it is up to you which model or models you choose to implement into your new facility. There is also a very popular hybrid version using all three types of training in one model. I am experimenting with this in my newest facility in Pennsylvania at this time.

So far I am enjoying the hybrid model, but I would not recommend it to the new business owner since you are dealing with all types of scheduling and space, plus equipment requirements.

Private Training

Pros: _____

_____

Cons: _____

_____

Semi-Private Training

Pros: _____

_____

Cons: _____

_____

Group Training

Pros: _____

_____

Cons: _____

_____

Hybrid Training

Pros: _____

_____

Cons: _____

_____

Final Selection

_____

② Create Your Program Ladders

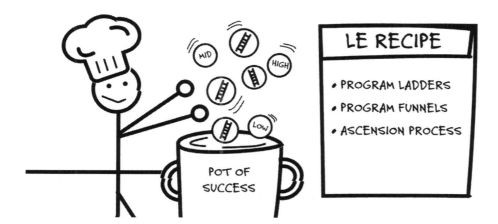

This is ingredient one in the secret sauce of your fitness business. Your program ladders are what will separate you from all other fitness business owners in your area. I have personally sold more than $3 million in fitness products programs and services using program ladders in all of my brands and businesses.

My program ladders allowed me to generate much more revenue than I would normally be able to generate because I could create pricing models based on intimacy and contact, rather than services provided.

If you replace the word "program" with intimacy or relationship you will understand program ladders in much better detail. Think about ways that you can create an integrated program suite that you can move your customer through so that they are continuously seeking higher levels of intimacy and contact with you, your brand, and your services.

Step one is to create the tier system and look at a common problem like belly fat, then create a tiered system of solutions ranging from low-intimacy to high-intimacy.

Let's look at an example. The magic key here is that every solution paves the way for the next level of intimacy while still being a complete program or product.

Problem: Women with belly fat left over from the first, second or third pregnancy that just won't go away no matter how much they diet.

- **Solution 1:** A free eBook that helps women isolate 10 foods that they should never eat if they want to get rid of belly fat once and for all. At the end of this book is a link to sign up for a free workshop on how to remove belly fat once and for all.

- **Solution 2:** The belly fat workshop discussed in the eBook, which is either given online or, better yet, in person every month at your facility. At the end of this workshop, the participants are offered a personal strategy session, a full body composition analysis, a custom meal plan and two weeks of a fat loss camp for $49 that is regularly $97.

- **Solution 3:** At the end of their second week of fat loss camp, the customer is offered a three-month pass to continue with their program for a discounted rate of $247, which is 40% less expensive than the current monthly rate. If they love the program, they do nothing and they can continue at three times a week during a specific time slot at the current rate of $147 a month when their three-month trial is complete.

- **Solution 4:** At the expiration of their three-month trial and as they are ready to sign up for the three-times-a-week option, you offer the "3X Wild Card" that gives them the ability to sign up for any time slots, up to three slots per week, for $197 a month.

- **Solution 5:** For a few extra bucks they get the added freedom of not being stuck in one time slot, so the 3X Wild Card may be a winner for those you never expected would be interested.

- **Solution 6:** You can also up-sell the customer into the unlimited "All Access" pass for $247 a month which gives them the ability to come as many times a week as they want, whenever there is an availability. This solution will be something that your biggest fans will gravitate toward because it gives them a chance to have more intimacy with your company, your trainers, and maybe you.

This is called a product ladder. This is how you should structure your fitness offerings so that you maximize revenue and build a tribe of loyal followers. They will always look forward to the chance to have more of you, and more freedom to pursue you when you frame it in a way that puts the highest level of solution against their most pressing problem.

Let's create your program ladders now if you have not already. If you have, let's look at how we can optimize them for potential income growth and customer retention by creating a class system that makes the lower class feel valued, but gives them something to ascend to, if they desire.

Tier 1 Program

What quick and easy solution to a specific problem could you offer a potential client that would help do these three things?

- **Solve** part of the client's problem and familiarize him/her with you and your brand.
- **Create** a sense of gratitude and a need for reciprocation.
- **Create** a desire for more of you and your higher-level services.

? — What program could you offer at the $0-$89 range that would solve an immediate problem your prospect faces, but still leave them wanting much more of you?

_____

_____

? — How will you deliver this in a powerful way that fosters a sense of gratitude for you and your brand so that your prospect definitely ascends to the next level of service?

_____

_____

? — How will you funnel your customer into the next tier effortlessly and seamlessly, so that they welcome the experience?

_____

_____

Tier 2 Program

What medium-value solution could you offer to your target market's most pressing problem that would also do these four things?

- Impress them with the level of effort you put forth.
- Make them feel like they received more value than their investment.
- Make them feel a strong bond with you and your brand.
- Make them want more of you.

? — What program could you offer in the $97-$297 range that would solve the core problem your customer faces but still leave them wanting more of you?

_____

_____

? — How will you deliver this in a powerful way that fosters a sense of gratitude for you and your brand so that your customer is likely to ascend to your next level of service?

_____

_____

? — How will you funnel your customer into the next tier effortlessly and seamlessly so that they welcome the experience?

_____

_____

Tier 3 Program

What high-value solutions can you offer to solve your customer's most nagging dilemma, and also do the following three things?

- Make them feel like an elite member of your family.

- Create a sense of pride in their decision to invest so deeply in you.

- Enhance an already strong bond between them and your brand.

- Make them want more.

? — What program could you offer in the $297-$697 range to not only solve the customer's core problem, but do it in a way that made them feel like it was done-for-them?

_____

_____

? — How will you deliver this in a powerful way that fosters a sense of gratitude toward you and your brand so that your customer is likely to maintain this high-tier service?

_____

_____

? — How will you funnel your customer into more exclusive offers effortlessly and seamlessly so that they welcome the experience?

_____

_____

Once you have mapped out your program line, you will need to create your pricing model so that you are getting prospects into your system with low barrier-to-entry products and programs and then ascending them to high levels of engagement and investment with your brand and your services.

3 — Numbers Forecasting & Income Goals

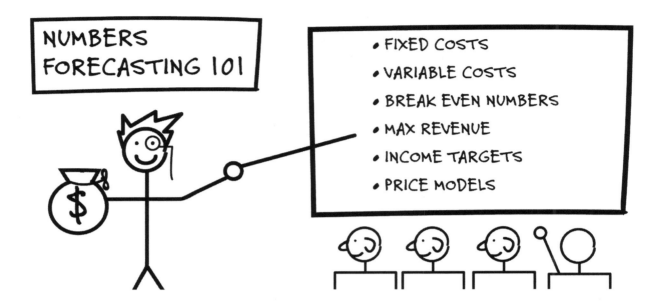

Pricing is important and needs to be done strategically. When setting your prices, always look at five things.

? — What are your fixed costs?

? — What is your break-even with your highest-tier program?

? — What is your maximum revenue with your highest-tier program?

? — What is your maximum revenue on your lowest-tier program?

? — How much net profit do you want to make in Year 1?

You do not have to have a lease or know what you are going to lease to do this. You just need a real estate agent to go over average lease rates in your city and the types of buildings available.

Then you decide where you want to start your business (in theory), and what those rates may be. It is really quite simple and can be accomplished with a single phone call.

Let's say for the sake of this book you wanted to start at around 1,500 square feet and the current annual rate was $12-per-square-foot. That rate included common area maintenance fees.

Your rent payment would be around $1,500 per month plus utilities, loan payments and liability insurance.

You can also determine your loan payments based on how much equipment you think you will need. A general rule of thumb is this:

Personal Training: $30,000 per 1,500 square feet

Group Fitness: $15,000 per 1,500 square feet

Right now the average loan payment on a $30,000 loan is around $500/month for 60 months. This is a great time to borrow money and hold onto your savings.

We know how much rent will be, and we know what kind of investment we will make (or the loan amount we will need). So it is time to validate our model and also set our pricing to give us a competitive starting point in the market.

Now we can validate our model and determine whether or not we have a winning business opportunity or we need to rethink our plan.

First we need to know our fixed costs. Here is an example of average fixed costs:

- Rent: $1,500
- Loan Payment: $450
- Electricity: $125
- Internet: $50
- Phone: $75
- Water/sewer: $65
- Insurance: $125

Total Fixed Costs: $2,390/month

Now we need to look at our break-even amounts. My highest tier membership is $497/month.

So my break-even is 4.8 members; let's call it five members in the high-tier program model.

After I get five members in my high-tier program, everything else that my business generates goes to my bottom line (minus payroll and miscellaneous expenses).

My lowest-tier program is $247/month so my break-even is 9.6, let's call it 10 members enrolled in my low-tier program.

Now I need to calculate my max revenue.

If I have 1,500 square feet and can be open six days a week from 6 a.m.-8 p.m. (84 hours per week available to generate revenue), I will need to figure out how much revenue I can make per hour.

As a general rule of thumb, you should reserve 300 square feet per private training session (2 people, trainer and client). You should reserve 125 square feet per group training client.

The most my facility can comfortably handle is five personal training sessions (1,500 square/feet divided by 300 sq/ft = 5) at one time, or one group training session of 12 people (1,500 square/feet divided by 125 square feet).

For the purpose of this exercise, I will assume we are doing exclusively personal training. Since each training session is 30 minutes, and five sessions can take place at one time, we can assume 10 training sessions can take place per hour. At the cost of $40 per training session, this means our max potential revenue per hour is $400.00 (10 x 40).

With 84 hours available to provide training sessions per week, I have the potential to generate $33,600 (84 x 400) in one week, $134,400 (33,600 x 4) in one month, and $1,612,800 (134,400 x 12) in one year.

The above figures reflect a 100% booked-solid business, which is highly unlikely, but gives me the peace of mind to know that, should I do that well, the structure and business model will support high revenue streams.

This is very important because you need to make sure that it is hard for you to outgrow the space based on your model, your numbers, and demographics.

To estimate an extremely realistic scenario, let's shoot low and assume that we are operating at 20% capacity for the first year.

Based on our max-revenue model, I can assume that my weekly gross revenue would be $6,720 (33,600 x 0.2), a monthly gross revenue of $26,880 (134,400 x 0.2), and a yearly gross revenue of $322,560 (1,612,800 x 0.2). Now don't get excited yet.

As an average, I pay out roughly 40% of my gross revenue to employees. This immediately leaves me with $193,536/year in adjusted gross revenue.

And let's not forget those pesky fixed expenses, totaling $28,680 (2,390 x 12), leaving $164,856 for our net profit.

Using this bare-bones financial breakdown, you can play with numbers confidently. The beauty of the small studio model such as ours is that at just 20% of max capacity, you can easily net six figures after just one year. Typical projections estimate a steady 10-20% growth per year, so I'll let you compute the profit margins in year 2, 3, 4, etc.

I can now say that I have done 3 things:

1 Validated my niche

2 Validated my market

3 Validated my model

Note: I recommend creating a pricing model that puts you at a break-even status with 5-10 members or less. You can always move to a bigger location if you outgrow your space, but small spaces can generate huge amounts of revenue while still feeling like a tight knit community.

I recently got my hair cut at a local salon and the place was literally packed. There must have been seven stylists working around me, all waiting room chairs and dryer chairs were full. The esthetician and two nail techs were also hard at work. I love business and I quickly calculated his hourly revenue to be more than $900.

His space was 1,400 square feet and their mortgage was under $1,000 a month. This dude was seriously killing it. He probably generates more than $100,000 a month in revenue. So I asked him if he was planning to expand to a larger location anytime soon, as he was busting at the seams. His response was "Hell no! I will stay small and take it all."

What a brilliant way to look at his business. It would be twice as much overhead, risk, and work to double the size of his business and there is no guarantee that the customers would respond well to more chairs and offerings. He is probably netting $600,000 per year and has few financial worries.

At what point do you say, "I am satisfied" and just enjoy life? Talking to him changed me a little and I am grateful for that change. I now have an income target and I will not try to reach much past it because more is not always better, even with money. Because at some point you will experience diminishing returns.

Create your pricing with a comfortable level of profit in mind and don't focus on becoming rich, because you will hit diminishing returns on the effort expended - the tipping point. Don't become a slave to insane goals and ideals for your business. Learn to be happy and find joy in the process, not the end result.

I was once told by a mentor to "never compare someone else's front stage with my own back stage. You should not look at others in the fitness industry and say "I want that life" until you know what their backstage looks like.

If they are getting up at 4:30 a.m. and not sleeping till midnight and never see their wife or family because they are too busy "killing it" to focus on anything else, they are already at a point of diminishing returns. Life is short and when you die you will not be looking back at income statements. You will be thinking about the people you love and the legacy you have left, if any.

Be the hairdresser, "stay small and take it all," and you will be happy, unless you know without a shadow of a doubt that you absolutely must be huge to be happy.

4 **Pricing Model Creation**

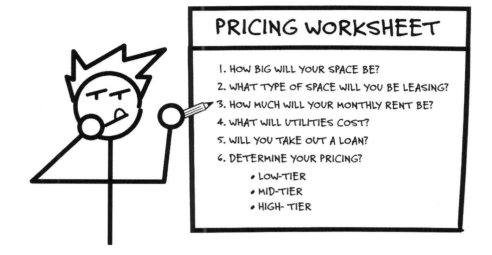

I think it is safe to say we have done enough due diligence at this point. We can now take the next step and strategically plan our fitness business.

Let's fill out your pricing worksheet:

? How big will your space be?

_____ Sq/Ft

? What type of space will you be leasing and what is the average price per square foot in your area for that type of space? Note: We will cover more on this in the site-selection portion of this manual. For the purposes of completing your pricing creation worksheet, please fill out the average prices for your local area.

Industrial _____ Per Sq/Ft

Light Industrial _____ Per Sq/Ft

Flex Space _____ Per Sq/Ft

Retail _____ Per Sq/Ft

Office _____ Per Sq/Ft

Medical _____ Per Sq/Ft

? — What is your monthly rent going to be, based on the fill-in answers?

(Size x Price Per-Square-Foot)

Sq/Ft X Price Per Sq/Ft _____

Add Extra Building (CAM) Fee _____

Divide total by 12 _____

Example:

1,500 X (12 + 3) = $22,500/ 12 = $1,875 per month.

So our base rent is $1,875 per month.

? — What do you typically pay for these utilities in your area? **Note: You can always contact the tenant of a space that is for rent and get the answers to most of these questions.**

Electricity _____

Internet _____

Phone _____

Water/sewer _____

Insurance _____

Trash _____

Totals _____

If you are going to take out a loan, place your estimated monthly payment on the line below.

Loan _____

By totaling the three amounts below you will have your total fixed costs, minus miscellaneous fees and payroll.

Rent _____

Utilities _____

Loans _____

Total Fixed Monthly Costs _____

? — What price point will you charge for your highest-tier monthly program so that 5-10 members enrolled in your program will cover your fixed operating costs?

Total Fixed Costs / 5 = _____

Total Fixed Costs / 6 = _____

Total Fixed Costs / 7 = _____

Total Fixed Costs / 8 = _____

Total Fixed Costs/ 9 = _____

Total Fixed Costs / 10 = _____

√ — Now find your pricing sweet spot for your high-tier program

High-Tier Program Price _____

? — What price point will you charge for your mid-tier monthly program so that 11-15 members enrolled in your program will cover your fixed operating costs?

Total Fixed Costs / 11 = _____

Total Fixed Costs / 12 = _____

Total Fixed Costs / 13 = _____

Total Fixed Costs / 14 = _____

Total Fixed Costs / 15 = _____

√ — Now find your pricing sweet spot for your mid-tier programs.

Mid-Tier Program Price _____

? — What price point will you charge for your low-tier monthly program so that 16-20 members enrolled in your program will cover your fixed operating costs?

Total Fixed Costs / 16 = _____

Total Fixed Costs / 17 = _____

Total Fixed Costs / 18 = _____

Total Fixed Costs / 19 = _____

Total Fixed Costs / 20 = _____

√ — Now find your pricing sweet spot for your low-tier programs.

Low-Tier Program Price _____

After completing this exercise, you will have a very deep understanding of what sort of monthly targets you need to set for growth and where your break-even points are for all your programs. This allows you to plan out your employee compensation structures with the confidence that you will always be able to add employees and expand your business without reaching a point of diminishing returns on your investment.

5 — Mapping Out Your Main Conversion Process

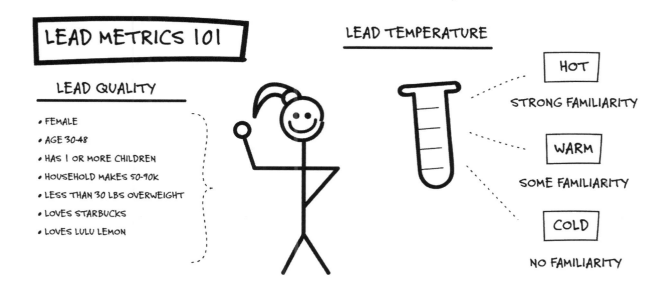

LEAD METRICS 101

LEAD QUALITY

- FEMALE
- AGE 30-48
- HAS 1 OR MORE CHILDREN
- HOUSEHOLD MAKES 50-90K
- LESS THAN 30 LBS OVERWEIGHT
- LOVES STARBUCKS
- LOVES LULU LEMON

LEAD TEMPERATURE

HOT — STRONG FAMILIARITY

WARM — SOME FAMILIARITY

COLD — NO FAMILIARITY

Your conversion process is one of the most important components of your business model and creating it requires your undivided attention. If you know what your conversion rate is on your conversion process, then you can scale your business just by the number of leads that cross your path. There are two factors that affect your conversion process on the front end.

- Lead quality
- Lead temperature

Lead quality is how closely your lead matches your ideal customer avatar that you created when you completed the niche selection and validation section of the launch formula. Let's say that your ideal market avatar looked something like this:

- Female
- Age 30-48
- Has 1 or more children
- Household makes 50-90K
- Is not more than 30 pounds overweight
- Loves Starbucks
- Loves LuLu Lemon

Now let's say you do targeted Facebook ads to this market using a social-scraping software program or just the Facebook ad wizard. You get 47 clicks to your offer using this targeting.

Your lead quality is excellent! You are attracting the right market to the front of your sales funnel and you have completed 50% of the lead equation.

You have just attracted 47 high-quality leads into your funnel.

The next thing we need to determine is the temperature of those leads. I use a three-pronged scale when determining lead temperature.

> **Cold:** Lead does not know you and is not familiar with your services.
>
> **Warm:** Lead knows of you and has heard about your services.
>
> **Hot:** Lead knows you, is quite familiar with your brand, and may or may not like you.

Now I want you to replace the word "lead" with the word "traffic." This is how your conversion process works.

Your conversion process is designed to take low-, medium- or high-quality traffic, whether it is cold, warm or hot, and convert that traffic into customers.

Your conversion process starts with something called a lead magnet. A lead magnet is simply a consumable medium like a checklist, workshop, process map etc... It has two purposes.

The first purpose is to develop a relationship with your prospect by giving something away that solves a problem, or moves them toward a compelling desire.

The job of the lead magnet is to get your prospect to want to take the next step with you. If this were an online conversion funnel, the next step would be to gather their email and permission to email them.

If this were an offline conversion funnel, then you would get your prospect to want to stay and talk to you after a workshop to get more information about your services and programs. We will dive deeper into the individual components of a conversion process later in this chapter.

But for now, just know that the conversion process starts with a lead magnet and ends with a person becoming a customer of your low-barrier offer, or in the best case scenario, a higher tier program.

It is a process and you need to have it thoroughly mapped out so you know how to create ads, create offers and move a prospect along your conversion process.

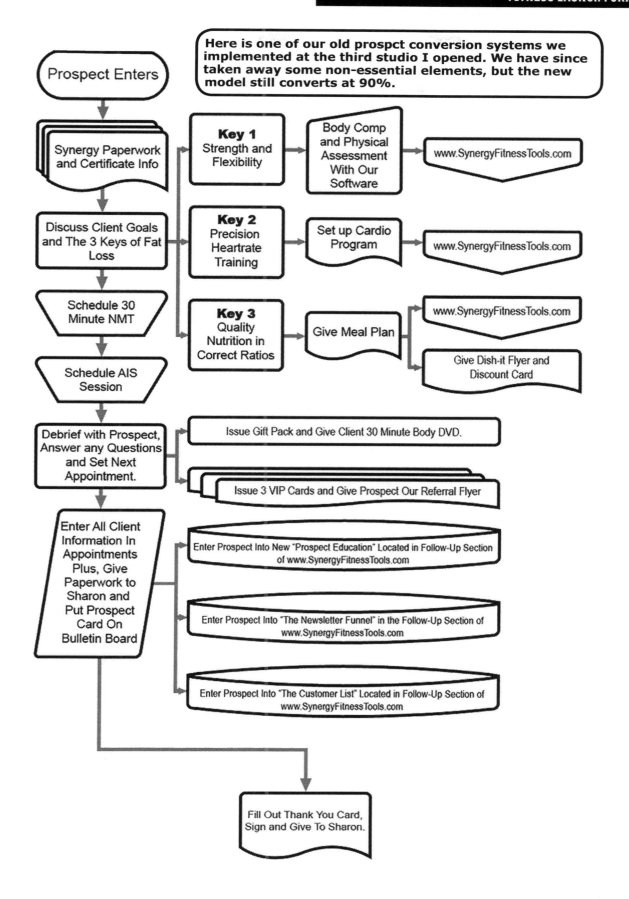

Here is one of our old prospct conversion systems we implemented at the third studio I opened. We have since taken away some non-essential elements, but the new model still converts at 90%.

Prospect Enters

Synergy Paperwork and Certificate Info

Discuss Client Goals and The 3 Keys of Fat Loss

Schedule 30 Minute NMT

Schedule AIS Session

Debrief with Prospect, Answer any Questions and Set Next Appointment.

Enter All Client Information In Appointments Plus, Give Paperwork to Sharon and Put Prospect Card On Bulletin Board

Key 1 Strength and Flexibility

Body Comp and Physical Assessment With Our Software

www.SynergyFitnessTools.com

Key 2 Precision Heartrate Training

Set up Cardio Program

www.SynergyFitnessTools.com

Key 3 Quality Nutrition in Correct Ratios

Give Meal Plan

www.SynergyFitnessTools.com

Give Dish-it Flyer and Discount Card

Issue Gift Pack and Give Client 30 Minute Body DVD.

Issue 3 VIP Cards and Give Prospect Our Referral Flyer

Enter Prospect Into New "Prospect Education" Located in Follow-Up Section of www.SynergyFitnessTools.com

Enter Prospect Into "The Newsletter Funnel" in the Follow-Up Section of www.SynergyFitnessTools.com

Enter Prospect Into "The Customer List" Located in Follow-Up Section of www.SynergyFitnessTools.com

Fill Out Thank You Card, Sign and Give To Sharon.

When mapping out your conversion process you should use 3-4 steps:

Step 1: The initial contact.

Step 2: The free version of and initial solution to a specific problem.

Step 3: A free version of your end solution that takes them one step further.

Step 4: A low-priced introduction to your core program.

Here is an example of a simple conversion process:

Step 1: Advertise on Facebook for a free workshop to increase vertical leap.

Step 2: Offer a free "jump mechanics review for each attendee" after the workshop.

Step 3: Review their mechanics, make suggestions for improving power, enroll them in an entry-level program.

Step 4: Escalate them to regular training after showing them a marked improvement.

Here is an example of an advanced conversion process:

Step 1: Target 30 females for a six-week female fat loss study that includes training and nutrition.

Step 2: Hold an orientation meeting and have them sign waivers and information releases.

Step 3: Document the entire process and get amazing results.

Step 4: Enroll the excited ladies in your core program for a discounted lifetime rate.

Step 5: Use all their before-and-after photos and testimonials to sell paid transformations.

Both conversion processes are well strategized and you can alter them to create hundreds of different variations to use to convert prospects to buyers. I recommend using one main conversion process for your offline funnels, and one main conversion process for your online funnels to get started. You can create a master conversion process that works for both traffic sources.

Use the worksheet on the previous page to map out your conversion process. Then I recommend going to **lucidchart.com** to input your conversion process into a more advanced process map to be used by you and future employees. You can store all strategy maps in your account and update them as you learn to tweak your funnels.

Let's map out your conversion process.

? — You offer what? Prospect does what?

You: _____

_____

Prospect: _____

_____

? — What is the next move you will make? What will your prospect do?

You: _____

_____

Prospect: _____

_____

? — What is the next move you will make? What will your prospect do?

You: _____

_____

Prospect: _____

_____

? — What is the next move you will make? What will your prospect do?

You: _____

_____

Prospect: _____

_____

? — What is your final move? What will your prospect do?

You: _____

_____

Prospect: _____

_____

Once you have the overarching strategy created for your conversion process, you will need to create your funnel maps. Your conversion process is the way you move a prospect through your sales funnel, but it is not an actual funnel.

Now that you know the way you intend to lead prospects through your funnels, you can now map out the process using the worksheet in the next chapter, then transfer your funnel maps to **lucidchart.com** for storage.

6 — **Map Out Your Funnels**

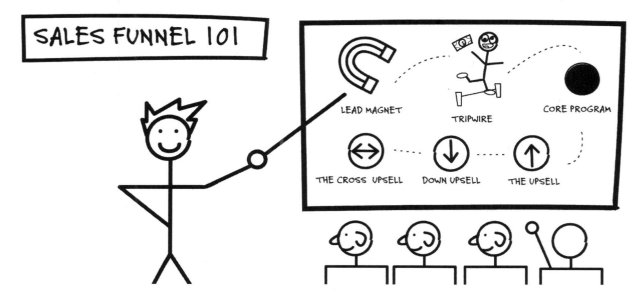

SALES FUNNEL 101

LEAD MAGNET · TRIPWIRE · CORE PROGRAM

THE CROSS UPSELL · DOWN UPSELL · THE UPSELL

A typical fitness sales funnel has about 3-6 stages and we will discuss them in detail in the following chapters. Here are the stages of successful sales funnels I have created with a few of my brands both online and offline.

> **Stage 1**: The Lead Magnet
> **Stage 2**: The Tripwire
> **Stage 3**: The Core Offer
> **Stage 4**: The Up-Sell
> **Stage 5**: The Down-Sell
> **Stage 6**: The Cross-Sell

Keep in mind that some of you may never have a need for stages 4, 5 or 6, but everyone will need to map out the first three stages if they want a successful funnel.

 If you want to get some advanced fitness sales funnel training please feel free to visit FitProEvolution.com after you open.

But in the meantime, we will cover two basic funnels you can use to open your new facility here in this book. Generally speaking, consumers will find you or come to know about you one of two ways:

This is great if you use these exposure sources in conjunction with a solid funnel that converts like crazy. But this is where most newbie fitness pros really screw up their marketing:

They trust that by getting their name out there they will get business. This is called hope marketing and it is what amateurs do.

What I'm going to teach you to do is drive prospects to your business through a series of strategically placed bread crumbs that lead them right to your front door and into your final conversion process.

Offline Exposure

- Referrals
- Drive-by
- Workshops
- Phone book
- Print ads
- Radio
- TV

Online Exposure

- Searches
- Your Website
- Newsletters
- Blogs
- PPC advertising
- Facebook ads
- Twitter tweets

Your Online Funnel

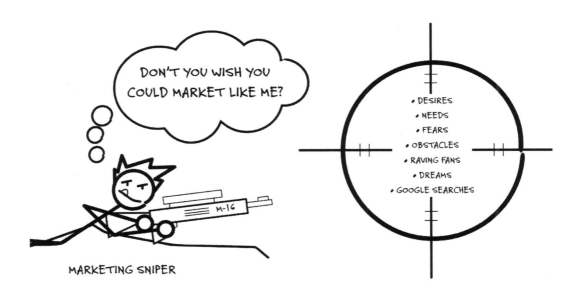

What could you offer someone browsing Facebook to make them want to investigate you further (only if they fell into your target market)? We discussed earlier that your avatar is what you want to attract, so what we need to do is make a list of things your avatar does.

Since our avatar is a woman who has children and is not totally deconditioned, we need to figure out two of the most powerful things that would cause her to take action.

Here are some things that make people take action.

- Something that can get them closer to a compelling desire
- Something that can get them out of, or away from a pain source
- Something they are preoccupied with or fear deeply
- Something that is an obstacle to their dream
- Something that they are huge fans of and want to consume more of
- Something they dream of becoming
- Something they obsessively Google

I asked my wife these questions since she fell into my target market, and these are the answers I received.

What is a compelling desire you have in regards to your health or fitness?

? To be completely toned, to have the energy I had as a teenager, and have a nutrient-dense diet.

? What pain or discomfort do you wish to eradicate or avoid?

The image that puts a bad taste in my mouth is of looking old, flabby and being too lethargic to move.

? What do you fear deeply about your health?

I fear that I could slowly let myself go and forget to re-evaluate myself along the way. I also fear the long-term effects of how I am treating my body now (by not sleeping enough, having high stress levels, etc.). I'm deeply afraid of cancer, and I know I could be treating myself better now to avoid some potential future cancer threats.

? What is your biggest obstacle to your dream?

My biggest obstacle is definitely time.

? What are you a huge fan of learning about?

Super foods that help defy the aging process, carcinogens, and the most effective, natural ways to stay energized.

? What do you dream of achieving or becoming?

I dream of a day where my major goals have been met, and I can make minor tweaks here and there but definitely have more free time to work out, and spend more time with family and friends.

? What do you obsessively Google in your free time?

I Google boots when I'm bored and too tired to dive into something heavy!

? What would you pay top dollar for in fitness?

I would pay good money to stay a consistent body fat percentage.

By asking my wife these seven simple questions I am able to create a lead magnet and trip-wire that she will most definitely be interested in consuming.

Here is a quick funnel I could put together that would definitely pique the interest of my wife based on her answers to my idea extraction questions:

1 **Lead Magnet:** Free tight-and-toned checklist and quick reference guide for women over 30.

2 **Tripwire:** The Tight & Toned 30-Day Makeover Metabolic Toning Camp for $67.

3 **Core Offering:** Unlimited training, nutrition and support for $147 per month (Guaranteed monthly body fat decrease).

4 **Up-Sell:** Night creams and supplements for age reduction.

5 **Down-Sell:** Online version she can do at home for $67 per month.

6 **Cross-Sell:** Time management workshops and organized mommy workshops.

Note: We will cover the details about setting up each section of your funnel in the following chapters. If you are stuck understanding a certain section of the funnel, you may read ahead so that you fully understand it before moving through the worksheet in this section.

Now it is time for you to map out your online and offline sales funnel. For the online funnels, I recommend that you use a **landing page software** and an **email auto responder service,** and I recommend a few great companies I use for this process on my resources page of my website.

 Here is a direct link: FitProEvolution.com/Resources

Bookmark this page, as I will refer you to it a lot so that you can get access to the best free and paid tools to get this launch formula completed with little or no headaches.

Your Online Sales Funnel Simplified

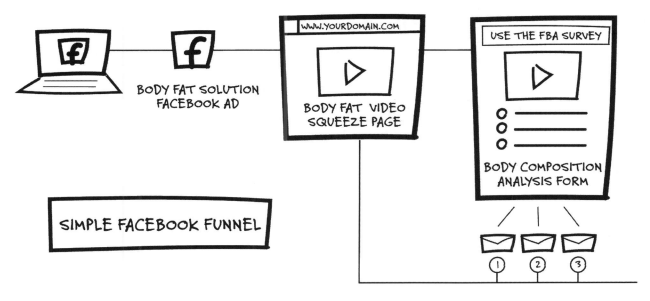

? — What avatar question will your lead magnet solve and what will the solution be?

Question: _____

_____

Solution: _____

_____

? — What avatar problem will your tripwire solve and what will the solution be?

Question: _____

_____

Solution: _____

_____

? — What avatar problem will your core offering solve and what will the solution be?

Question: _____

_____

Solution: _____

_____

? — What avatar problem will your up-sell solve and what will the solution be?

Question: _____

_____

Solution: _____

_____

? — What avatar problem will your down-sell solve and what will the solution be?

Question:_____

_____

Solution: _____

_____

? — What avatar problem will your cross-sell solve and what will the solution be?

Question:_____

_____

Solution: _____

_____

We will refine this later using lucidchart.com, but for now you have a very basic understanding of how you will convert cold traffic into paying customers using this online sales funnel (which you will create later during the launch process).

Don't worry if this section feels overwhelming. I have broken down two of my best converting funnels in this book, but if you'd like to seek exactly how to get these funnels up and running smoothly, and you can find out more about it in the resources section of my website at **BrianDevlin.com/Resources**

Let's move into your offline sales funnel now and map out the components that we will create later in the launch process when we actually build our business. Offline sales are a little different than online sales and usually the traffic is slightly warmer and easier to convince. For offline funnels, I recommend driving traffic to a live event or live workshop.

Sometimes a phone call is effective too. Offline funnels thrive when people are able to meet you in person and get to know you in a no-pressure environment. It is much easier for them to develop an affinity for who you are and what you do when they can see you in person.

Use the following worksheet to map out your offline funnel.

Your Offline Sales Funnel Simplified

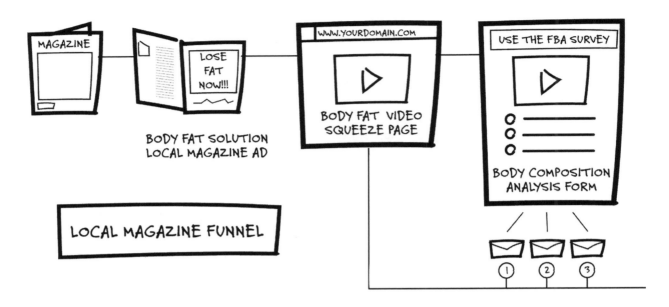

? — What avatar question will your lead magnet solve and what will the solution be?

Question: _____

_____

Solution: _____

_____

? — What avatar problem will your tripwire solve and what will the solution be?

Question: _____

_____

Solution: _____

_____

? — What avatar problem will your core offering solve and what will the solution be?

Question: _____

_____

Solution: _____

_____

? — What avatar problem will your up-sell solve and what will the solution be?

Question: _____

_____

Solution: _____

_____

? — What avatar problem will your down-sell solve and what will the solution be?

Question:_____

_____

Solution: _____

_____

? — What avatar problem will your cross-sell solve and what will the solution be?

Question:_____

_____

Solution: _____

_____

⑦ Creating Your Lead Magnets

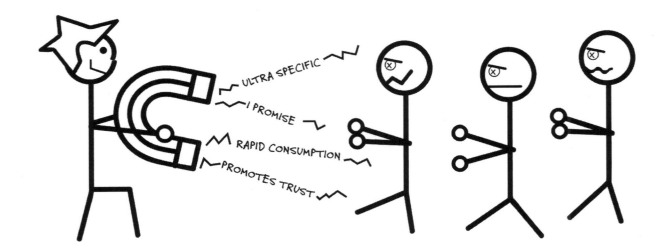

Your sales funnel starts with something called a lead magnet. A lead magnet is something that piques the curiosity of your target audience. The prospect feels an overwhelming need to consume whatever quick solution you are offering.

An online lead magnet is usually presented in the form of an opt-in page or landing page. Your prospect reaches this page through a Facebook ad, a Google AdWords campaign, a banner on a popular local site, or just a plain old internet search.

These are usually keyword-specific pages that offer a solution to one big problem, and the prospect is drawn into your funnel usually through a compelling headline or anchor statement.

Example: Facebook News feed ad with a picture of a mom in a pushup position with her child sitting on her back and a headline that says, **"Find out how this stay-at-home mom was able to lose 4 dress sizes and fit back in her skinny jeans in 36 days. Download the same action plan she used to do it right here!**

There is a specific image and headline you would use for this ad that would appeal to your target audience. In the Facebook ad creation wizard, you would target females age 28-48 that lived within 10 miles of your city. You could also target specific interests such as Starbucks coffee, LuLuLemon, athletic clothing.

When the prospect clicks on this ad because it piques her interest, Facebook will redirect her to something called a squeeze page. Here is where you would have a professionally designed landing page that offers a solution to the same problem but gives a nice visual image.

 This is an example of a landing page that converts well: FitnessLaunchChecklist.com

Here are the rules you must follow when creating your lead magnet:

1 Your lead magnet must be ultra-specific in nature. You can't solve a vague problem. It has to capture the reader's attention and keep it. "Find out how this stay-at-home mom was able to lose 4 dress sizes and fit back in her skinny jeans in 36 days. Download the same action plan she used to do it right here!"

Here is an example of something you would not want to use. "Find out how anyone in the world can improve their overall health and feel great!""

This is too vague and will not pique the interest of a specific avatar.

2 Your lead magnet must solve one immediate problem quickly. This is important to remember. You want to offer something that the lead wants right now and will consume immediately. They want the action guide!

3 Your lead magnet should have one big promise attached to it. In this case you are delivering an action plan that will help a woman lose 4 dress sizes in 36 days.

4 A lead magnet removes barriers. If that action plan were $39, you would not convert the prospect into a subscriber because they don't trust you yet.

5 Your lead magnet is designed to promote trust. When a lead gets your action plan, the plan needs to live up to its name and be a valuable piece of literature that can be used effectively. This will foster trust.

6 Your lead magnet must have a high perceived value. Your consumer should feel like they would pay money to get this information. You are delivering an 'aha' moment to them free of charge. This promotes likability.

7 Your lead magnet must be designed for rapid consumption. A good rule of thumb is:

- **Online lead magnet:** Should be able to consume it completely before their coffee cup is empty.

- **Offline lead magnet:** Should be no longer than 45 minutes if presenting to a captive audience.

When your lead magnet is rapidly consumable to an audience, when it costs nothing to consume, and provides a real world value that gives the prospect a definite 'aha' moment, she will desire more of you because you have just anchored three vital emotions in her head.

- **Familiarity** with you, your brand and your authority.
- **Likability** for you and your teaching style.
- **Trust** in you, your brand and your future products, programs and services.

When these three emotions are present, you won't even have to ask for her to take the next step. She will be asking you for your services without you having to "sell" anything.

What I am illustrating here is not some cutting-edge sales NLP or conversion voodoo. It is simply the act of making friends. Look at the age old "cup of sugar" example. Your neighbor is making a pie and is missing a vital ingredient. You get a knock on your door. Not only do you oblige your neighbor, but you throw in your grandmother's secret recipe for apple tarts that you know is amazing.

Your neighbor comes back a week or two later just raving about those tarts and wants to know if you have any other goodies in your recipe box for cookies., following it up with, "I owe you one!"

You now have fostered with your neighbor these three elements:

- Likability
- Familiarity
- Trust

Your neighbor likes you now and wants to do nice things for you like watch your kids in a pinch or share a famous lasagna recipe with you. You have just added a member to your tribe, and if you need anything in the future you've got it with no questions.

The same holds true with your lead magnet. The headline is the cup of sugar. The secret tart recipe solves the problem in a bigger way.

Now that you know what you need to magnetically attract your customer, let's create some lead magnets!

Lead Magnet Creation Worksheet

? — What ultra-specific problem of your prospect are you solving?

_____

_____

? — What big promise will you deliver with your lead magnet?

_____

_____

? — What barrier to the sale will you overcome with this lead magnet? (Price, time, level of investment)

_____

_____

? — How will you build trust with your prospect through the use of this lead magnet?

_____

_____

? — How will you elevate the perceived value of this lead magnet through its construction?

_____

_____

? — How will you design this for rapid consumption leaving the user wanting more of your high-value solutions to their urgent problems or compelling desires?

_____

_____

? — How will you prime your prospects for the next stage in your funnel and lead them to consume your tripwire, or core offering, with enthusiasm?

_____

_____

Once you have mapped out your lead magnet, I recommend you use the outsourcing resources listed on my resources page at FitProEvolution.com/Resources/

These are the same providers I use to get work done, hire virtual assistants, find qualified designers, writers and do the things that move my businesses forward.

8 — **Create Your Tripwires**

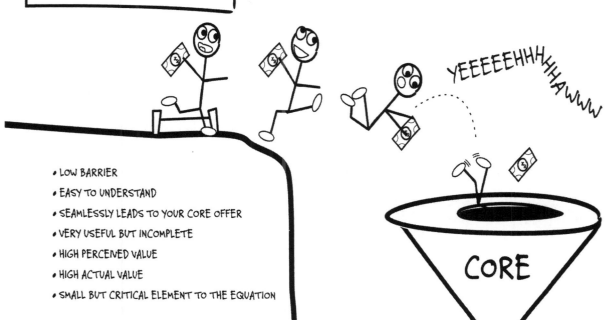

EFFECTIVE TRIPWIRE

- LOW BARRIER
- EASY TO UNDERSTAND
- SEAMLESSLY LEADS TO YOUR CORE OFFER
- VERY USEFUL BUT INCOMPLETE
- HIGH PERCEIVED VALUE
- HIGH ACTUAL VALUE
- SMALL BUT CRITICAL ELEMENT TO THE EQUATION

YEEEEEHHHHHHAWWW

CORE

Your tripwire is what causes your prospect to set off the conversion land mine. Simply put, it is what makes your prospect think they like you, know you and trust you enough to actually give you their business.

There are some very important rules that must be followed when creating tripwires in order for them to be effective and create high conversion rates.

In war, a tripwire is attached to a land mine, snare or some other hidden object that will cause death. If the enemy just placed a giant bomb in the middle of a path, most soldiers would just avoid that area and continue on.

Your tripwire is the same way. It camouflages the awkward process of doing business with a complete stranger.

This is not to be confused with deception or trickery. You are selling a product that your customer needs but, unfortunately, because of the horrible advertising practices used on most consumers, their guard is already up when it comes to honest service providers.

So we use the tripwire to break the prospect's initial resistance to purchasing from us by lessening the financial blow, and over-delivering on value. Another term we could use is "Welcome Mat" if it makes you feel better.

The key to remember when designing your tripwire is that it needs to be a low-barrier offer, usually meaning low in price or commitment.

Here are the requirements for crafting an effective tripwire for your funnel.

- Low barrier
- Easy to understand
- Seamlessly leads to your core offer
- Very useful but incomplete
- High perceived value
- High actual value
- Small but critical element to the equation

Knowing that the tripwire is similar, but a step above, the lead magnet, we can now create an effective tripwire for our core offering using the criteria above.

A poor example of a tripwire would be the typical half-off your first month of training, because it not only devalues the core offer, but it is not incomplete. If your group training program is your core offering, then offering half-off the core offering will do nothing except devalue your core program.

Unfortunately, that is how most fitness businesses go about doing business and attracting customers into their offering. Groupon is a perfect example of this.

A great example of an effective tripwire would be to offer your prospects a total body assessment and movement screen and create a map of everything they should focus on if they wanted to work out by themselves in a gym without you. Give this to them for a 90% discount if they take action within the next 48 hours.

Here's why:

- The offer is low-barrier as it does not cost much
- The process is easy to understand
- It is very useful, but incomplete without a guided workout program (your core offering)
- It is a small, but critical element of the equation
- It has a high perceived value because it is a scientific assessment
- It has a high actual value because it requires your expertise and interpretation
- It can seamlessly lead to your core offer

Now that you understand the psychology and requirements behind an effective tripwire, please create your own tripwire for your funnel by using the worksheet below.

Tripwire Creation Worksheet

? — What low-cost, high-value solution can I offer my prospect immediately after they consume my lead magnet?

_____

_____

? — How can I make this offer simple to digest and easy to understand?

_____

_____

? — How can I make this offer very useful and attractive, yet still incomplete?

_____

_____

? — How will I craft this service or product to seamlessly lead my customer to my core offer and then up my program ladder?

_____

_____

? — In what format will I deliver this service or program so that it is rapidly and enthusiastically consumed?

_____

_____

? — What tools or services will I need to get this completed quickly and on budget?

_____

_____

If you need help outsourcing this process or setting up the tools required, please see my resources page at FitProEvolution.com/Resources. I reveal almost all the tools I use on a daily basis on that page for your convenience.

Once your tripwire is complete and you have your funnel components in place, you can move on to your groundwork strategy.

CHAPTER SIX

The Groundwork Begins

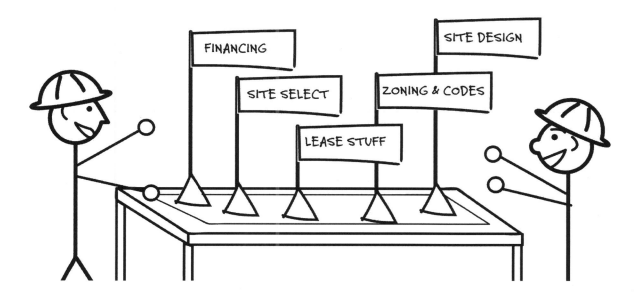

OK, welcome to the groundwork section of this formula. This is where we are going to roll up our sleeves and dive into this venture with both feet and here is why:

There is no guesswork involved anymore. We have deeply developed our brand. We have validated our niche and market. We know our estimated break-even numbers and our estimated fixed costs. We know how we are going to magnetically attract our leads and turn them into customers. We know how we are going to ascend those customers to fully devoted followers of our fitness brand.

I can borrow money with confidence at this point and continue checking items off my list. Fear should never be a factor at this point because we have a seriously solid plan. I have opened a bare-bones fitness business from scratch with just my savings account and I have opened a top-of-the-line-facility using the bank's money. My personal opinion is that you should keep your money and use the bank's money. At the time this book is being written, business bank loans are as low as 3%-4% and cap at around 5.8%.

My last facility was built with just a $30,000 loan at 4.8% interest. So basically for a car payment, you can open an awesome facility.

1 — Create Your Business Entity

After you have decided on your name, you will need to do a search on your state or province's website to make sure someone else does not have your desired name. You will be able to tell in minutes if you can file the paperwork needed to create your business entity. Check with your local Secretary of State. It takes five minutes to find out if a name is taken in your state in most cases and it is free. Once you have a green light with the state, see if you can reserve the dot com version of your business name for your website. This is not super-important, but helps when new prospects have heard about you and they type your name into Google later on.

Next you need to decide if you are going to be one of the entities listed below.

- Sole Proprietor
- Limited Liability Company
- Limited Liability Partnership
- Corporation
- Sub-chapter S Corporation

There are other entities you could form, but I will not be discussing them in this book. I do recommend speaking with your accountant before making a final decision and filing your final articles of incorporation.

Find a quick article that details everything you need to know about entity types and the pros and cons of each: FitProEvolution.com/Resources/

I recommend also that you fax, not mail your articles of incorporation to your Secretary of State. If you have an attorney, it is helpful for them to review your final articles before submitting them because most states will return your articles and reject your request if you so much as miss a capital letter or a suffix. They are extremely strict in what they will accept, so a good legal review is advised before submission.

My first attempt at incorporating by myself was a three-month process with three consecutive rejections for simple grammar errors. I hope you benefit from my mistakes. Make sure you also make a copy of your submitted articles because most banks will require them for a commercial account to be created. Sometimes a business entity requires state seals for approval, but with a little sugar and playing dumb, you can speed up the process by giving the bank a copy of your *submitted* articles, and they may start your business account ahead of time.

Next you will need to acquire financing and this is actually much easier than you think. You just need to be organized before you go out asking for money.

(2) Time to Acquire Financing

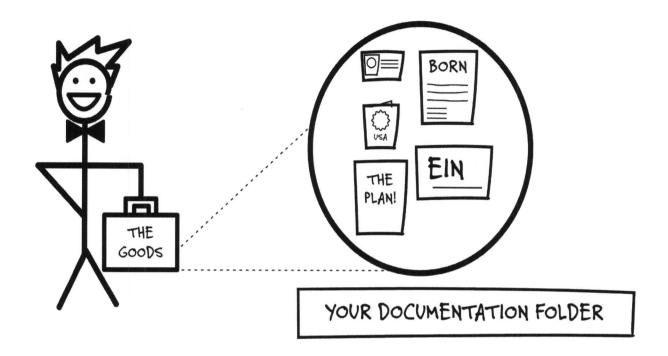

YOUR DOCUMENTATION FOLDER

The easy way: Make a list of 10 banks in your area, compile a portfolio with documents listed below, dress nicely and get 5-10 quotes for a local business loan. Banks want to support local business and they will encourage you to bank with them once you are up and running. You will need:

- Driver's license
- Birth certificate
- EIN or Social Security number
- Passport
- The last three years' tax returns
- A record of all your assets or personal income statement
- Business plan if you have one (just a few paragraphs may be all you need)
- Articles of incorporation or receipt of processing
- A few local utility bills for record of residence

You may need a few more documents and a few more IRS forms, but seriously you can get most of it within a day. I recommend keeping a folder with all this stuff in one place in a file cabinet or a safe.

When you have all these items, you will be able to do many things quickly and efficiently such as:

- Lease a company vehicle
- Get utilities turned on
- Create your business bank accounts
- Get lines of credit
- Negotiate a commercial lease
- Talk with the zoning office
- Talk with the code office

This folder will make quick work of the rest of your tasks if you keep it organized and keep adding to it as you encounter a new need.

After you negotiate with the banks and you find a good loan amount, make sure you get a few things clear before signing the commercial loan.

- What is the interest and how is it compounded?
- What is the term of the loan?
- What is the total payoff amount?
- What is the total interest paid over the course of the loan in a specified dollar amount?
- What are your monthly payments and are they fixed or variable?
- What are the pre-payment penalties, if any, attached to this loan?
- What happens if your loan is sold to another lender?
- What sort of extra filing might underwriting request? Example:: UCC 118 Filing

After you have the green light for your financing, you will need to start looking at real estate to rent or buy, depending on your business model.

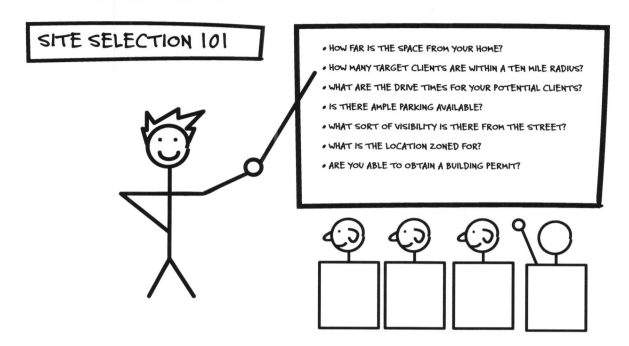

③ **Site Selection Process**

OK, now that we have a solid business idea and model put together, it's time to see if we can actually find a space that meets all our needs. This is the part that can be the most frustrating, because your business is now in the hands of fate and the local real estate market. All too often, fitness pros make the mistake of renting or leasing a space that does not fit the needs of their business or their model, and they end up pulling their hair out trying to make the venture work. I have done this.

The purpose of this section is to help you make an educated and healthy decision before negotiating your terms and signing a lease.

Here are seven very important factors in determining where to lease space.

? — How far is the space from your home?

This is actually a very big factor. It is important that your facility is close to your home. If you have to drive 35 minutes to reach your facility every day, that is going to put more than an hour of drive time on your car and kill an hour of time you cannot use productively, aside from listening to self-improvement CDs during the commute. All three of my facilities were less than a five-minute drive to my home and I did this strategically so I could maximize productivity and damage control if an employee decided not to show up for a session.

My newest facility is walking distance to my house and I can't tell you how awesome it is to run home for lunch or take a walk down to do some work on the weekends. It is so, so, so nice!

I fill up the tank on my car about once every two weeks because I have strategically designed my life and lifestyle to support human powered travel or very short drives. Not all of us have this luxury, but we can learn to be selective based on what it is we really want.

? — How many members of your target market live within 10 square miles of your potential facility location?

This is a vital piece of your site-selection puzzle. Most people will not drive more than 15 minutes to go to a fitness facility. Yes there are outliers, but we don't play the risk game with my system. We play the strategic game. Make sure that there are at least 10,000 members of your target market within 10 square miles of your facility. If you were to attract just 1% of those members, you would have at least 100 members and your break-even would be between 5 and 20 members.

To find out how many members of your target market are living within 10 square miles of your proposed facility you can use demographic search companies like Info USA and other demographic data sites for businesses. You can even use their mapping tools to draw a 10-mile perimeter around your proposed location and purchase a list of all the members in your target demographic. You can then send test campaigns to these members directing them to a "coming soon" squeeze page to see how many hits you get with a bulk mailing or postcard.This is a rather extreme version of being strategic, but I have done it with success in the past.

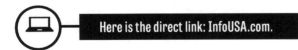

Here is the direct link: InfoUSA.com.

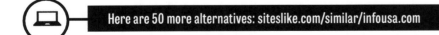

Here are 50 more alternatives: siteslike.com/similar/infousa.com

? — What are the drive times for potential clients to your proposed location? What kinds of obstacles will your clients encounter on the way?

Drive times are very important and something you need to look into if you live in metropolitan areas.

Because of land structures like mountains and rivers, drive times can be severely affected even when a location is within 10 miles of your target market. Make sure to create a list of any traffic obstructions or busy areas that could seriously affect drive times to your proposed location. Also pay attention to city planning and new road construction by attending your local government meetings prior to leasing space in any suspect areas.

? — Does your proposed location offer enough parking for your members if you were to grow quickly?

One of the biggest mistakes I ever made was setting up my second gym in a location where parking was ultimately going to become an issue, and it did. We were forced to relocate after five years because the landlord decided we took up too many spaces and the new restaurant was getting upset.

Since the restaurant was willing to sign a 15-year lease, I was indirectly forced to leave by way of a massive rent increase strategically enforced by our landlord. This was all because I did not ask questions about the parking when I signed the initial lease in 2008.

Don't settle for limited parking!

Remember, ease of access is another very important factor when thinking about parking. Don't lease spaces that are a pain to get in and out of, because you will just upset your members and they will eventually go somewhere easier to navigate and park.

? — What kind of visibility and traffic does your proposed location have?

Believe it or not, this is not as important for fitness businesses because we grow more from referrals and not walk-ins. But visibility and traffic is always nice to have. The thing you need to stay focused on is the cost of that visibility and traffic. Most high-visibility and high-traffic lease locations are more expensive than those off the beaten path, and actually offer far less opportunity to expand if needed.

Sometimes the less-visible locations can be leased for a steal and offer limitless opportunities for expansion and redesign.

The group fitness businesses that are cult-oriented fare very well in low-visibility areas, but if you wanted to open up a boutique fitness studio where you were attracting a more affluent market, I would consider traffic and visibility when choosing your potential site.

? — What is your proposed location zoned for?

This is one of those super-important elements that a lot of fitness pros don't know about or understand. Zoning can make or break your ability to open up a fitness business. It varies by state and city, but each state, province and city has zoning offices where you can dig into the nitty-gritty of zoning law and find out if your proposed location will encounter rolls of "red tape" when you try to start construction or obtain a building permit.

I found a perfect location for a medium-sized transformation center in my home town and almost signed a letter of intent on the building, which happened to be an old tire repair garage. It had a perfect location, tons of traffic, ease of access, roll up doors, cement floors, 15-foot ceilings, ample parking and office space built into the location. It was reasonably priced at $8 per square foot and was 3,500 square feet.

I literally would have just had to paint and do a few light construction elements to the bathrooms and we would have been ready to go.

So I called the zoning office and they informed me that it was zoned "stateside terrace," which was some 100-year-old zoning classification that came with a 175-page stipulation manual and it would require legal fees and lots of time to get the area rezoned.

Had I not asked this question and called my local zoning office, I would never have known that after signing a lease and trying to obtain a building permit, my life would have beome extremely difficult trying to get the zoning changed while eating up all my free rent.

Make sure your proposed location is zoned for a fitness center or able to be rezoned without problems.

? — Can you get a building permit? What will it really take?

In a lot of states and provinces, getting a building permit is the same as getting a business license, meaning that you cannot get a certificate of occupancy without getting a building permit and going through the entire process of plumbing, electrical, building, and fire inspections. This is required even if you have no planned structural changes, which can be quite frustrating and time-consuming.

What I have found to work best is to go to the code office in your area and let them know that zoning is approved for your type of fitness business, and that you want to know what you will have to do to pass codes in your area before you sign a lease.

Townships thrive on income generated by local businesses, so they need your business. And if you are honest about your intentions and let them know what your areas of non-negotiation are (meaning what it will take for you to bag the idea and walk away), most code offices will give you some sort of variances, as long as it will not affect the safety of your future patrons.

My township code officer was very harsh and fatalistic in my initial meeting with him and I looked him in the eye and said, "I'm getting the feeling that you don't want me to open the doors. Is that true?" He said "Absolutely not! We want nothing more than for you to succeed, but we have a job to do and we will not compromise safety for your convenience."

I simply replied, "I would never want or ask you to, but what I do want is to open the doors without spending my life savings because, quite honestly, the way you are framing things, I am fearful that I will not be able to afford this business here."

What he said next was what made me realize that it did not have to be so hard. He said, "You know, you can always appeal anything I say to you."

That's exactly what I did. I appealed most of his requirements with valid reasons why they were not appropriate or necessary. Seven days later, I won my appeal. Now, most people would have quit right there when the code officer was talking about adding bathrooms and ventilation systems, wheelchair lifts and all sorts of unnecessary building requirements.

That's what they want you to do. They only want fighters to have businesses, because fighters stay open when quitters close the doors. Business turnover is not good for the local economy and the code offices are there to see that only the fittest survive the tests. But you can use due process to stay the course even when you don't have the budget of big businesses in similar pursuit.

Meet with your code office and get a signed list of all your requirements before signing a lease so that you don't have to battle all this through the free rent period. You will be very glad you did.

4 — Visit the Code Office

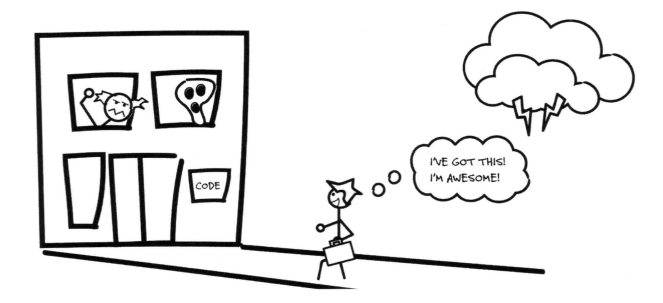

Before you sign your lease or even begin the negotiation period, you should plan a trip to the code office to meet with the local building inspector. This can be a very stressful experience.

You will most likely find the staff very stern and not interested in any small talk. You will be treated as if you do not matter. If members of the code office have to repeat themselves, it can become ugly very quickly, so I recommend you be prepared when embarking on this adventure and not enter into it blindly.

If you think the office staff are bad, wait until the actual code officer comes out to see you. He will act like you have no reason to be there and make it seem as if you are wasting his time by breathing.

But now you know, and you can prepare accordingly. Code officers are people. People like to be respected, listened to and affirmed. The biggest thing you need to remember is respect. These are the same guys that meet with Walmart developers and they have seen a lot of stuff.

Give them the respect they deserve. Call them sir or ma'am and don't argue with them. Let them be heard. Act dumb and be patient. They will eventually relax when they see that you are not there for a fight, and are determined to get a business opened.

Some items you should bring with you:

- Renderings of the proposed space (Get copies from the landlord)
- A site plan of what you want the facility to look like
- A list of questions you want to ask
- A copy of the current zoning document
- Pictures of the parking lot
- Pictures of the inside of the building
- Pictures of the stuff you want to change (walls, doors, etc.)
- Receipt from the zoning office (request to change zoning)
- Signage renderings
- ID
- Checkbook

Questions To Ask At The Code Office:

? — Will I need to do any ADA upgrades?

Usually if you are doing any sort of build-out or structural change to your existing space, a percentage needs to go toward handicap-accessible upgrades, and these can be quite expensive. So know your rights concerning ADA laws in your area.

? — Will I need to do any electrical service upgrades?

When my wife and I opened our first and second chiropractic offices, we had to upgrade the electrical service to a 200-amp service. This cost thousands of dollars and we had to get new electrical system architectural renderings. After hiring an electrician and a board-certified architect, we added $3,000 to our opening costs.

? — Will I need to do any plumbing upgrades?

Most fitness facilities will be required to have an ADA-certified, dual-basin water fountain if your occupancy limits are more than 15 patrons. These can be purchased online for under $1,000 and can be installed for about $400. Make sure you know these requirements, and hire a plumber whose price includes getting you to pass code.

? — Will I need to get architectural renderings and seals?

Any time you make structural changes, the building inspector can request that you get architectural renderings prior to commencing construction. It has been my experience that an architect usually charges $300 an hour and renderings are not cheap. Definitely use your appeal power to get past this if you can. If they are required, confirm that it will be sufficient for the new renderings to cover only the areas where change will be made. You may be required to have complete new renderings of the entire facility, but by playing nice, you might be able to twist the arm of your inspector and drastically reduce architect fees.

? — Will I be required to install sprinkler systems or fire-suppression systems in my fitness facility?

Most landlords have had to do this already if the space is big enough for a bunch of occupants or stored goods in order to suppress catastrophic fires. Sometime you will find a location that failed to add fire suppression and this may be something the code office requires. Never pay for fire suppression. Always negotiate that with your landlord, as it should be their responsibility.

Once your lease is signed, you have no recourse. I made the mistake of renting a massage studio space back in 2003, and hired a plumber to put in a shower so massage clients could go right from the table to the warm shower.

Great idea in theory. Well the building inspector had a field day with my operation and he made me install a sprinkler system, fireproof material and emergency lighting all in a one-room studio with a clear exit. That mistake cost me $2,000, but I learned from it. And now I can save you the heartache of getting bullied by a building inspector, because you will have a signed letter from the code office stating what is actually required ahead of time.

? — Will I need a traffic study?

Sometimes with high-volume businesses like boot camps, local code offices will require traffic studies to be completed before letting you open a business. These are expensive and should be avoided at all costs. The requirement may even involve changing your business model.

? — Can you provide a detailed list of what I will need to get my C/O?

Most code officers will complain when you ask this question, but they are required to give you the facts as they pertain to your situation and are state employees who have supervisors.

Now I definitely do not recommend ruffling the feathers of your local code officer, but you should be able to get a detailed list of everything you need to get your certificate of occupancy during your initial site inspection.

THE TEN COMMANDMENTS

THOU SHALT ALWAYS HAVE A RENEWAL OPTION

THOU SHALT ALWAYS TRY TO GET FREE RENT.

THOU SHALT ALWAYS TRY TO GET A TERMINATION CLAUSE

THOU SHALT ALWAYS GET A RIGHT TO SUBLEASE

THOU SHALT NOT BE RESPONSIBLE TO THE ANCHOR TENANT

OF LEASE NEGOTIATION

THOU SHALT NOT BE UNINFORMED ABOUT THE LANDLORD'S SIDE DEALS

THOU SHALT HAVE YOUR BANKER REVIEW THE LEASE

THOU SHALT NOT SIGN AN "AS IS" LEASE

THOU SHALT CLARIFY WHO MAKES REPAIRS TO YOUR PROPERTY

THOU SHALT READ THE LEASE IN ITS ENTIRETY AND LEASE DOLLAR PRODUCTIVE SPACE

Congratulations! You are actually doing this. Take a minute and pat yourself on the back because this is a milestone few people have reached in the fitness industry. Not only have you researched, blueprinted, validated and tested your business idea, you have also jumped through the hardest hoops you will ever have to handle.

I would be lying if I told you the rest was easy, but I can honestly say the rest is fun, empowering and life-changing.

So before we get started I want to mention that I have used an attorney to negotiate every lease I have ever signed. The job of an attorney is to find areas where you are vulnerable and negotiate a more fair arrangement. I do not recommend negotiating a commercial lease without an attorney. Don't be cheap. A good attorney will cost you between $250 and $500 to negotiate your lease.

Here is my lease negotiation hot list. These are things that you may not think about until it is too late and you are left holding the bag.

Most of these items of discussion are lessons I've learned in my 15 years of business. These were hard lessons I will help you avoid learning the hard way. They were, and still are painful!

The 10 Commandments of Lease Negotiation

1 Thou shalt always have a renewal option.

Never sign a commercial lease without a renewal option even if you have no plans of being there in five years. Always have at least two renewal options in place. Don't ever take a landlord's word for it. Everything must be in writing. You never know what is going to happen. Try selling a business with no lease. It's like trying to sell air. Never leave yourself open to losing your business regardless of your plans to be in a location long term. Always have an out. Always have an option.

2 Thou shalt always try to get free rent.

When you do things right with the blueprinting, validating and testing of your business model and you build your business before signing a lease, you have much more freedom. While most gym owners burn through their free rent getting through code, waiting on equipment and setting up systems, you will be able to open the doors shortly after signing the lease and in most cases recoup your loan payments before actual rent even commences. I have done this and it was awesome. There will always be unforeseen headaches, but in most three-year leases, you can negotiate six months of free rent upfront. You may have to pay CAM fees, but at least your overhead for months 1-6 will be so low that you can pay back a huge percentage of your loans and start-up costs before it gets real.

3 Thou shalt always try to get a termination clause.

Some landlords will allow you to have some sort of termination or max-liability clause in your lease that protects you from the landlord accelerating the lease and holding you accountable for the lease legally in the event your business does not make it. Nothing is worse than going out of business and having a landlord sue you for an empty space. I don't expect that this will ever happen to you, but it could and it is better to be prepared for the worst-case scenario. A termination clause could limit you to only paying a few months of the lease after you vacate, as opposed to paying for the remaining 18 months. You will likely be able to negotiate a termination clause or max-damages clause if the property has been on the market for a few years and the landlord is eager to rent it. I was able to negotiate a six-month termination clause on my last space, and never did have to use it.

4 Thou shalt always get a right to sublease.

Some leases don't allow subletting or subleasing. Avoid signing these. They severely restrict your ability to exercise options and grow your business. At one point I had 10 sub-lessors in one of my locations and they netted me a lot of extra cash. Make sure you have this option.

5 Thou shalt not be responsible to the anchor tenant.

Make sure your landlord discloses any and all side agreements they may have with the anchor tenant. Many times, property owners are so desperate to get the large spaces rented that they will give anchor tenants special rights of refusal and privileges. If the anchor tenant won't agree in writing to give you quiet enjoyment rights within your space, then don't sign the lease.

6 Thou shalt not be uninformed about the landlord's side deals.

Make sure the landlord discloses any and all side deals they may have with other businesses in the local area. Those deals could affect you and lead the landlord to impose unlawful restrictions on your business. These would not hold up in court, but other businesses could take you to court and tie you up in litigation attempting to enforce a prior written agreement.

7 Thou shalt have your banker review the lease.

Your loan may require this to protect you in case of default. Which will allow you to assign the lease to another tenant instead of being sued for damages without recourse.

8 Thou shalt not sign an "as is" lease.

Never do it. If you sign an "as is" lease you literally have zero recourse against anything that could happen to your property.

- If the facility floods, you pay.
- If it gets hit by lightning, you pay.
- If it needs repairs, you do them.

Landlords will try the "as is" lease if they sense a potential renter is running out of time with their search or they have potential tenants fighting over a space.

9 Thou shalt clarify who makes repairs to your property.

Clarify who must cover the cost of maintenance, repairs and other common property expenses. If the owner or management company covers these costs, ask for the specifics. If you have to cover them, ask for a cap on the amount that you must pay so that the owner will cover any maintenance costs above that threshold.

10 Thou shalt read the lease in its entirety and lease dollar-productive space.

Look at the cost of the lease, and determine whether it is a total cost for the property or if it is on a per-square-foot basis. If the cost is per-square-foot, inspect the property to see if it has space you can't use, and ask that the landlord remove any unusable square footage like closets, bathrooms and so forth.

Check for any area covering rent escalation over the course of the lease. Ask that landlord include an escalation clause to prevent unexpected increases. Finally, make sure you read the lease in full and have your attorney read it for any concerning areas that may not be in your best interest to sign or may be unlawful.

6 — Complete Your Initial Site Inspection

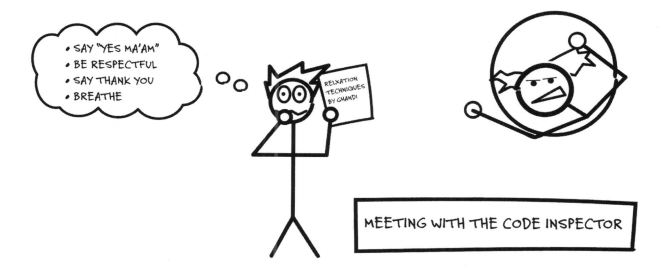

MEETING WITH THE CODE INSPECTOR

After you finalize your lease and you have access to your new space, you will need to obtain a building permit in most states and provinces, regardless of your intent to modify the structure.

This will be kicked off with your initial site inspection, where a local building inspector from the code office will show up at your facility location and insist on seeing anything and everything in the building. You will most likely be treated poorly and condescended to. Fight the urge to react.

Never, and I repeat never, speak disrespectfully to one of these inspectors. They are all in high-stress, high-volume jobs and they absolutely won't tolerate it. Losing your cool with a building inspector will definitely hold up your project and cost you thousands in extra work.

- Is it right? No.
- Is it fair? No.
- Is it just? No.
- Is it going to change? Probably not.
- Is it reality? Yes!

Since I would rather open businesses and thrive than fight with a building inspector, I do three things when they come around:

Nod and say "yes sir/ma'am" to everything they say.

Act dumb yet respectful when they ask questions.

Thank them for showing you the clear path.

If you do this, your projects will go much more smoothly and you will open much faster. Most building inspectors will show leniency when given respect and affirmation. They also get nicer as you move through each step of inspections, because they start to recognize your capacity for being the 10%.

Remember, when you don't agree with something, file a formal appeal and use the process. It usually only takes a few days to hear back from the director. Do not bring it up to the inspector on site. Not a good idea.

You should now have a list of code requirements (rough and final inspection items) you will need to address while building out your space, if any. If there is no build-out required, usually you will need to make some sort of ADA upgrades or add ADA water fountains and bathroom fixtures, if your building does not already have them.

Here is a list of common items the code office may request of a fitness facility:

- Fire suppression system (Negotiate this with landlord as it is a deal breaker financially for you)

- ADA water fountains (usually around $1,400 with install)

- ADA bathroom upgrades and wheelchair turning radius requirements (Negotiate with landlord. Very expensive)

- Adequate ventilation (You are not mercantile so you may have stricter requirements)

Your next step is to draft your facility renderings and compile your master lists. Let's do it!

7 Designing Your Facility Layout

I have a secret weapon when it comes to facility layout and I have created a unique training video to show you exactly how I designed one of my facilities. Using this, you will see that in just a few hours you can see exactly how much equipment you should order, how much money to borrow, and the steps required to turn your self-made rendering into a reality.

 Go to FitProEvolution.com/Resources/ (Click the facility design training link)

This is a detailed video showing how I created my facility in Charleston, S.C. You can have special access to the tool I use to get the best results. I think you are really going to enjoy this bonus training!

Before watching this free training, pay attention to the six action items below that you will need to focus on when designing your facility for optimum effectiveness and client satisfaction.

- Client flow (Will customers feel crowded or is there plenty of open space?)
- Equipment layout (Same as above)
- Organization (Try to keep things off the floor when creating storage options)
- Visual clutter (What will your customers see, smooth clean lines or equipment stacked everywhere?)
- Overall artistic expression
- Using paint and mirrors

Enjoy the training and good luck with your facility design!

8 — Compiling Your Master Lists

I really enjoy this part of the launch process. This is where you get to take the facility layout you desire to create and make it a reality. You get to finally see your dream come to fruition as soon as the list is complete.

You will need four lists.

1 Your build-out or structural change list

- Materials list
- Labor list
- Price sheet

2 Your large equipment list

- Large pieces of equipment
- Analysis equipment
- Flooring
- Cable machines
- Plate loaded machines
- Selectorized machines
- Dumbbells
- Plates
- Bumpers
- Collars
- Kettle bells
- Olympic bars
- Pull-up rigs
- Slide board
- GHD
- Plyo boxes
- Equipment with a lead time of greater than two weeks

3 Your small equipment list

- Bands
- Balance cushions
- TRX
- Pull-Up assisters
- Mats
- Medicine balls
- Slam balls
- Wall balls
- Equipment with a two-week lead time or less

4 Office equipment list

- Bathroom supplies
- Computer
- Check-in software
- Payment processor
- Scheduling software
- Office supplies
- Sound system
- All the stuff you need that has a two-week lead time or less

Once you have your lists compiled, just create a Google spreadsheet with columns that look like this:

Equipment | Date Ordered | Date Received | Problems or Notes | Quantity | Cost Each | Total Cost |

Create a page for each section and you can share this directly with your accountant who can create a depreciation sheet for your corporate tax returns.

You can use strike-out text or a certain color fill when each item is completed so you can easily track and share information about your opening with your team.

9 — Finding Skilled Labor for Your Build-Out
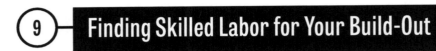

I do not recommend hiring a general contractor to get work done. I use local handymen, plumbers, flooring installers and so on. When hiring local labor, I use a few web sites and ask friends and family for good referrals. Usually I can find a good provider in an afternoon.

Here is a little test I do with all the providers I hire. I start by asking them if they have ever done commercial work that was inspected by the code office. If they say no, I am done right there. Never hire a provider that has not worked with building inspectors. You will most likely regret the outcome.

Next, I ask them if they are good at passing code with their work and they usually reply that they don't usually have any problems. After they say this, I say "awesome, so I am going to give you one price for this job and that price includes any and all changes you will have to make to appease the building inspector."

This separates real skilled labor from the talkers. If they are OK with this, I give them a $100-$200 small job to do and I walk away. If that job is done without any problems, I usually hire the contractor. If they have a bunch of questions, make excuses about finishing tomorrow or anything else, I'm done with them.

First I post on my timeline that I am looking for a good service provider on my personal Facebook page. I ask people to PM me only. I usually get some great leads from this.

 Next I use the two sites I have listed in my resources section at FitProEvolution. com/resources/ (Click on the local service providers section).

Good luck finding your contractor. I am confident those tips will save you some serious money.

CHAPTER SEVEN

The Build

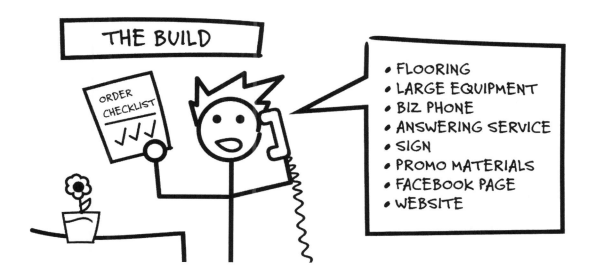

At this point, we have obtained our building permit, had our initial site inspection and have a list of code requirements. We have probably found, interviewed and hired a few service providers for any projects or build-outs we need done, and we have started marking items off our launch lists. Now we can focus on the engineering and completion of everything we need to open on time and with a professional edge. Let's get started!

1 — Select And Order Your Flooring If Any Is Needed

Flooring makes a space usable and attractive and there are all different looks and feels of flooring you can use. I have used wood, rolled rubber, polished cement, martial arts flooring and interlocking tiles in my facilities and I would have to say they all have certain pros and cons.

Wood

Pros: Looks great, is great for bodyweight stuff and yoga, and you can use sliders. It holds up for years.

Cons: Easily damaged with weights, and you can't use sleds. It is not comfortable to lay on, and is susceptible to water damage.

Turf

Pros: Looks great, is sled compatible, and you can lay on it. It is durable, great for groups, and great for body weight.

Cons: It is hard for Olympic lifts and difficult to clean.

Rolled & Interlocking Rubber

Pros: Excellent for almost everything.

Cons: Not sled-compatible.

Martial Arts:

Pros: Super comfortable and easy to clean; great for yoga and body weight.

Cons: Easily damaged by shoe traffic, as heels go through it; weights damage it and it is not sled-compatible.

I recommend ordering the flooring early, as the lead time on it can be as much as a month and you can't move in any equipment or set anything up until the flooring is installed.

Don't make this mistake either: Do not install flooring until your drywall and any work that involves power tools is complete. Make sure all the dust is cleaned up.

Timing your flooring is paramount to success. It needs to be well-organized or you will be left with a plethora of problems you don't want to deal with.

I have included a few links to flooring companies I have used with good service and decent quality at competitive rates in the resources section of my website.

 You can see them here FitProEvolution.com/Resources/. Click on the flooring providers links if you want to see who I use.

Once you have the flooring ordered, you should start ordering your large pieces of equipment. We will cover this next.

② Ordering Large Equipment Pieces

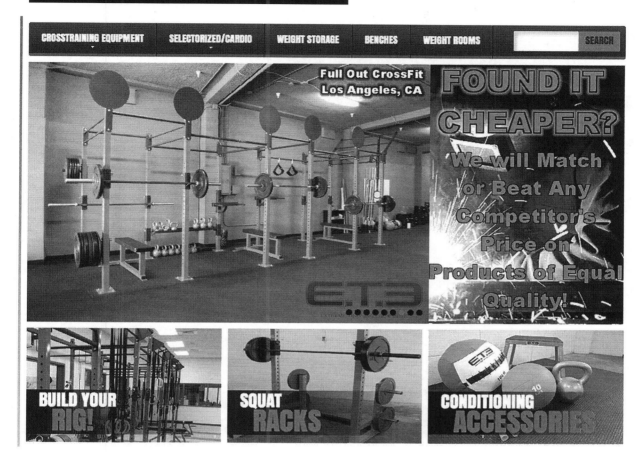

Ordering large pieces of equipment like pull-up rigs, squat racks, dumbbells, kettle bells and so forth can be very invigorating and was one of my favorite parts of the launch process.

But there are some key things you need to take into consideration before you order your large equipment.Here is a list of questions I would ask before placing an order on any large equipment pieces.

? — Do I have double doors at my facility that we could bring a pallet full of equipment through, or will it have to be broken down outside and carried in?

? — Is the building accessible from the street for a dolly, and are there cutaways in the curbs outside for delivery, or will I have to take equipment off the pallet just to get it over the curb?

? — Could a large delivery vehicle get into my parking lot and close enough to my building to make a freight delivery?

? — Will I need extra help getting this shipment in the building and unpacked? If so, make a list of 10 people you could barter with for help, or hire someone.

? — Will my delivery vehicle have a lift gate or will I be responsible for getting the pallet or boxes off the truck myself? (Get this in writing)

? — Is this piece of equipment in stock or is it manufactured after I place the order?

? — Does this piece ship assembled on a pallet with shrink wrap or does it come in pieces or boxes and I have to put it together?

? — Have I checked for bad reviews and screened the vendor and transport company prior to placing an order?

? — Do I have a guaranteed delivery date with recourse for failure to deliver on time, and "damage free" in writing?

? — Do I have adequate ceiling height for the piece I am requesting? Make sure you get all the specs, including the weight of the piece in question.

? — What sort of shipping precautions are taken to avoid damage to my equipment? What is the damage policy?

This list of pre-order questions should save you hours and hours of headaches when it comes to getting your large equipment ordered and in the building on time, damage free.

When your order does come, here are some key points to remember when receiving a delivery.

√ — Always unwrap and check the shipment fully for damage before signing the bill of lading.

√ — Take inventory of the entire shipment and compare it with the freight manifest.

√ — Take pictures of how the pallet was secured in the truck and the condition of the shrink wrap.

√ — Take pictures of any damage, even scratches. Photograph the entire order.

✓ — Always write "Subject To Inspection" on the Bill of Lading when you sign your name.

✓ — Take as long as you need to feel good about your order. The driver is paid to wait.

✓ — If you are not comfortable with an order, refuse it. Never accept an order you are dissatisfied with.

We complete the equipment orders early so we have time to correct course if there's a problem.

To see a list of the companies I use and more resources about ordering large equipment, please see the resources section of my site at FitProEvolution.com/Resources.

Let's keep moving. Opening day is fast approaching and there is still a lot of work to do. But don't worry, I've got you covered. We have a proven launch formula.

3 — Establish Your Company Phone Number

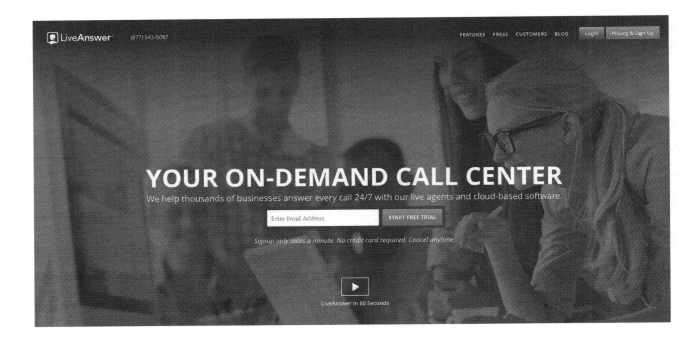

You have a big decision today. Do you use your cellphone as your company phone number, get a professional number linked to an answering service, or get a local phone number with a phone and answering machine inside your facility? Either way, you can't really move forward with your signage or promotional materials until you have a phone number to place on them. So you will need to get this taken care of sooner rather than later.

Here are my thoughts. I have used all three options and I will never again rely on a local phone number or cellphone for the following reasons:

- I only want to talk to prospects when I call them.
- I don't like being caught off guard and discussing business when I'm not prepared or in the mood.
- I don't like caller ID blocking.
- I like to make return calls at certain times of the day.
- An answering service is trained to get the information you need before the prospect hangs up.
- An answering service is more professional in my opinion.
- An answering service weeds out telemarketers who will relentlessly call your cell and business phones.
- An answering service answers the phone every time it rings. You won't.

Now you know how I feel, but you still need to make your own decision. I have included a list of providers I have used, and still use, in the resources section of my website.

If you decide to go with an answering service, here are some keys to selecting the best service for your investment.

1 Make sure you can keep the number if you leave the service. Some companies will try to keep your phone number. This is not legal in most states, but make sure you check and read their written policy on this. You have a lot invested in signage and promotional material using that number.

2 Listen to their clients and check for reviews on non-affiliated sites before you sign any agreements.

3 Avoid companies who want you to sign a long-term agreement up front. Month-to-month companies are usually more reputable because they have no reason to trap you into business with harsh contract penalties.

4 Make sure your calls are not outsourced to the Philippines, India or any county that is known for massive call center services. You want callers to feel like they could be talking to someone locally, not in another country.

5 Have a satisfaction guarantee and be sure you have the freedom to dictate exactly how the provider will answer the phone and what they will say. You may pay more for this feature, but you want the option to be available. If it is not, choose another provider.

6 Test your service completely and have at least five friends or family members call and attempt to play different customer roles. Don't put that number on your promotional materials until you are completely satisfied with the process.

I hope you have an easy and smooth experience getting your phone situation set up. Next, we will need to get our signage designed, approved and on the building as quickly as possible. You will want to attract customers and let people know you will be opening weeks, or even months, before you actually do.

4 — Designing, Approving And Ordering Your Signage

Let's be honest. You can get swindled trying to get a sign on your building. The sign companies are high-profit businesses and they charge a premium because people expect to pay it. I am of the mindset that less is more, and my signs never cost me more than $1,000 installed.

Here are a few ways to save money on your sign. Remember, you can always redesign your sign later. My personal philosophy is that once people start to hear about you, your brand, your amazing team and your professional business, they won't remember your sign as anything more than a landmark showing where you are located.

You can design your sign yourself, or get a simple text logo put together and make that into a sign. My signs are very simple and so are my logos. Simplicity always trumps loud obnoxious advertising in my opinion. Look at my book cover. It is simple and the promise is simple. *"The no fear, no b.s., no hype, action plan for launching a profitable fitness business in 60 days or less – from someone who's done it."* The book has one promise, 2 fonts and 3 colors. It is attractive to the right audience and was simple to create.

One of my signs says:

> *Synergy Fitness: Advanced fitness training and neuromuscular therapy*

Another Says:

> *Synergy Fitness: Advanced fitness training and corrective exercise*

The signs are simple and on painted sign board, with my three company colors: red, black and steel. Play around with some simple sign ideas. Once you find one you like, go get it approved by your landlord, and then get it approved by your local zoning office.

Here are some things to remember that will help your sign get approved quickly:

- Use a sign that won't cause the public to complain. If they don't like your sign, they won't like your business.
- Use colors that won't clash with your building.
- Know the measurements of your proposed sign idea ahead of time.
- Know where the sign will go and have Photoshopped renderings of the sign in your folder.
- Know which direction your sign faces.
- Know the tax parcel number of your sign's location.
- Make sure you have a final proof of the sign in your folder.

Remember, you can always change your signage. Some companies use vinyl banners for the first few months they are in business, then get signs made after their grand opening. The most important thing is to get your sign approved and on the building or roadside monument so you can let the public know you are coming soon!

For some helpful tools and design companies I use, please see my resources page at FitProEvolution.com/Resources.

Next we will want to create your Facebook fan page and design your promotional items — and this may be easier than you think!

5 Creating Your Facebook Fan Page

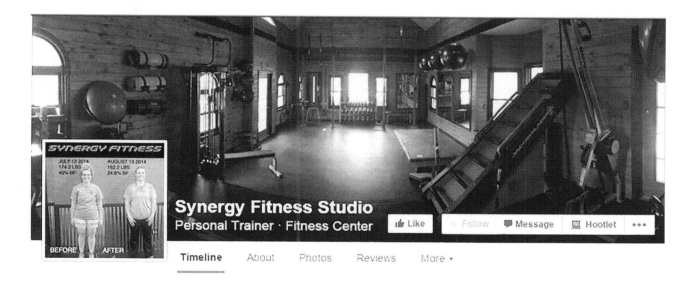

I'm not going to dive deep into the science of creating the perfect fan page, and I teach much more about this topic in my **Fitness Launch Academy** program.

You can learn more about joining our community at FitnessLaunchAcademy.com.

Your fan page is the epicenter of your marketing message, and you should post relevant content on your Facebook fan page to help your visitor achieve a goal or solve a problem they may have. Your fan page is where you can display all your reviews, testimonials, before-and-after photos and more.

I use my fan pages to drive prospects to our live events and our free consultations. It is very effective if you want to capture an audience and over-deliver value while still driving them through your marketing funnel. Most of my lead magnets originate on either my fan page or through Facebook targeting.

Here are some elements you should definitely have on your fan page:

- Company information and hours
- Company website
- Reviews
- Posts highlighting member achievement
- Cool branded info-graphics and diagrams
- Branded relevant photos
- Recipes
- New studies
- Challenges
- Tips, tricks and tactics for staying fit

Remember, your fan page is your brand and it needs to interact seamlessly with your website. A visitor should not feel any sense of disconnect when they leave your fan page and head over to your company website. Make sure there is some level of expectation and consistency between the two.

I have also posted some tools for enhancing your fan page performance in the resources section of my website.

Next we need to get our promotional materials designed, and these too need to be consistent with our website, fan page and look and feel of our facility.

6 Designing And Ordering Promotional Materials

I recommend starting your promotional materials with a one-page, two-sided flyer. It's difficult to understand what to put on a flyer, because there are so many snippets of information about your company you could use. But I have a different approach. I design my flyers like a long-page sales letter. I start with something called a white paper and have a designer turn that into a super-attractive, effective flyer. Remember, your flyer is also part of your funnel and needs to be designed as such. It is drawing them to either your lead magnet, tripwire or core offering, and should have your call to action embedded in many ways.

I also recommend giving up on business cards and instead using plastic gift cards that contain a redeemable gift the prospect or receiver can use immediately. Why would you hand someone a business card so they can throw it where all their other business cards go? Most people throw business cards on their dresser when they get home and empty their pockets. They sit for a few days, then are swept into the trash when the clutter in their room is removed.

In my **Fitness Launch Academy** coaching program, I walk you step-by-step through this process and give you the actual PDFs of all my promotional materials and signage. Feel free to check it out for a deeper understanding of promotional material design. Here are a few key points you need to cover when designing your flyers and gift cards:

- Who are you and what do you do.
- What are your services and how can they help.
- What do typical results look like.
- Who has used your services with success.
- What sort of time requirement is involved.
- What is the general price range for your services.
- Why are you qualified to offer your services.
- Who is your program for, and who is it not designed to serve.
- One specific call to action.

Your gift cards should offer a specific gift and one way to claim the gift. I recommend just leading the prospect to your answering service on all promotional materials. My philosophy is all funnels lead to the answering service or a consultation request form.

I would never put an email address or a personal phone number on any promotional materials or sales funnel stages. You want all your leads to go to one or two end points and that's it. Keep it simple and don't make your funnels complicated. More hoops = fewer conversions.

7 Design & Launch Your 'Coming Soon' Page

This process can be easy or complicated. With landing-page software, this may take 30 minutes maximum, and you will be finished and collecting leads.

If you use a designer, it may look better, but will take up to a week to finalize and get up on the web and visible. Your "coming soon" page is very important because it helps you build that valuable prospect email list.

This page also tells visitors who you are and approximately when you will be opening. But it also can be linked to your pre-sale strategy. You could have a "coming soon" page that allows a prospect to get on the email list for your notifications. That allows you to market continually to them until they either come in, unsubscribe or just add your email address to their spam filter.

I go deeply into the psychology, design and implementation of landing pages, coming soon pages, sales funnels and conversion voodoo in my coaching program **Fitness Launch Academy.**

 I have also included some landing page software resources I use in the resources section of my website FitProEvolution.com/Resources.

Feel free to check out either of the above resources.

Here are some key points to adhere to when designing your "coming soon" page:

- Use a two-step opt-in page with a progress bar on the second step
- Craft a compelling headline that will make the visitor want to get your updates
- Keep the opt-in button on the first screen. Don't make the viewer scroll to find it
- Keep the page clutter-free and use clean lines
- Make the page all about one simple thing: Getting updates about your opening
- Link the page with an auto-responder that will allow you to broadcast to people on the list
- Set up a five-day email series that educates the prospect about your brand and the benefits of your services

OK, now host your landing page on a keyword-specific domain like ChicagoBodyTransformations.com, or host it on a back page of your site like YourDomain.com/Coming soon.

Both options work, but make sure you have analytics installed on all your pages. This way you know the conversion rate of your opt-in or "coming soon" page.

Analytics will show you how many came to your site, where they came from, how they found you and whether or not they clicked anything or just left your page.

The data will help you optimize your page for the highest rate of conversion. This is marketing gold! Do you realize a simple 10 percent increase in opt-ins on your page could net you tens of thousands in more business?

What's even crazier is that a massive client influx could come from changing a few words, an image or a button color.

Imagine making an extra 25K-40K this year because you increased your funnel opt-ins by 10%. All you need to do is look at analytics and some heat maps, make a few changes and that's it!

I cover all these tricks in my coaching program, **Fitness Launch Academy**, but I also have some analytic tools you can use in the resources section of my website.

Next we need to order our printed material, as it has a decent lead time from receiving a proof to the day it gets delivered.

8 — Order All Printed Promotional Material

When you are ready to get all your promotional materials ordered, you can do it one of two ways. You can use an online service or you can do it locally. Both options have pros and cons.

Usually the online print-on-demand companies are cheaper, but the lead time can be up to four weeks for a box of flyers. Local printers are usually more expensive, but can have your materials in just a few days.

I use different online sources for:

- Flyers
- Postcards
- Door hangers
- Gift cards
- Clothing
- Towels
- Water bottles
- Bracelets
- Vinyl signs and banners
- Yard signs
- Stand up banners

I list a few of them in the resources section of my website FitProEvolution.com/Resources, and all of them in my coaching program FitnessLaunchAcademy.com.

It's good to get these items ordered and in circulation early so you have more exposure for your grand opening.

We will cover more of the groundwork items in the next chapter when we discuss tweaking and polishing our offerings and methodically getting our business ready for our dry-run training in Phase 6 of the formula.

CHAPTER EIGHT

Tweaking And Polishing

1 — **Setting Up Your CRM System**

A CRM system is a customer relationship management platform. In my opinion, it is imperative for you to have this incorporated into your business from the start. Remember, your business is all about relationships and acquiring your customer's continued loyalty every month with the currency of service. When your customer has solid expectations of you and you have solid expectations of your customer, your relationship is a breeze to engage in. If there are blurred lines and communication is poor, you will quickly find yourself with resentful customers. Watch your attrition rates soar!

The job of your CRM is to become the automatic liaison between you and your customer. Its sole purpose is to get your message to their ears and eyes quickly and reliably. Here is how our CRM software, FBA, works (also see diagram on next page):

- It delivers the meal plans I use
- It delivers the cardio programs I use
- It delivers the messages I need to send with a few clicks and no typing
- It integrates with Mindbody, our scheduling and payment-processing system
- It tracks email open rates by customer
- It sends surveys to my customers
- It sends videos to my customers
- It requests testimonials from my customers
- It requests and rewards my customers for referrals
- It delivers company updates and policy changes
- It delivers birthday and "thank you" messages
- It saves me hours each week
- It allows me to create niche audiences and send targeted promotions my other customers can't see
- It is mobile responsive

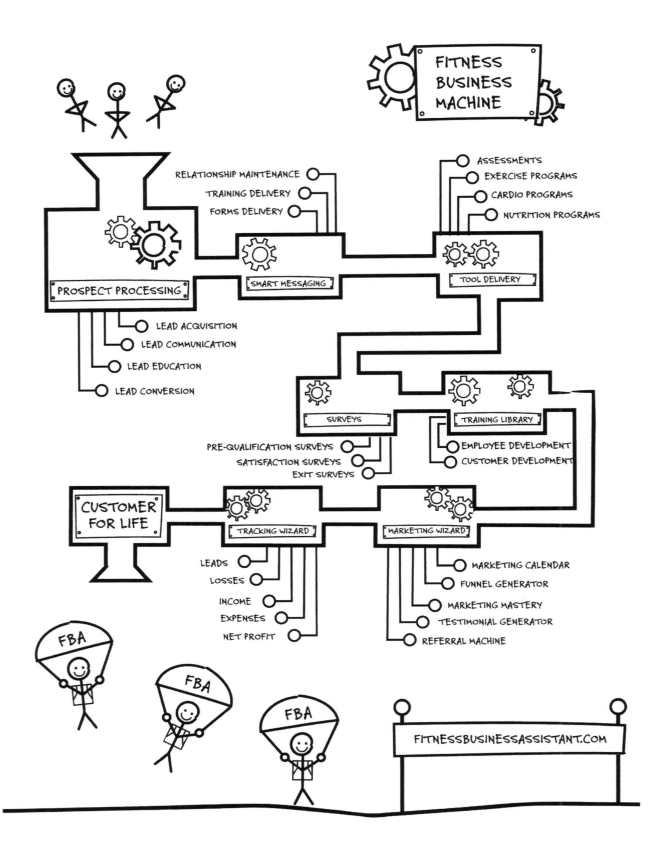

There are some very important questions you need to ask yourself as you build your CRM system. I will cover eight of them here.

When putting together your CRM program and creating your "FBA Smart Messages," you need to ask vital questions to craft the process and path you will use to move your customer through your program ladder.

? — Does my customer feel understood?

? — Does my customer feel heard?

? — Does my customer feel that I care about them?

? — Does my customer feel generously served?

? — Does my customer feel at home and like they belong here?

? — Does my customer feel a strong sense of structure here?

? — Does my customer understand my expectations?

? — Does my customer feel educated?

We use our CRM system to achieve these ends through surveys and strategic contact, simplifying and automating the process of keeping customers happy. It is much easier than you think and my **Fitness Launch Academy** program gives you access to all our CRM systems and how we use FBA to run our company.

The biggest way to satisfy your fitness customers is to wow them with your programming and equipment quality.

 You can find some of the program-creation resources and equipment providers I use in the resources section of my website FitProEvolution.com/Resources/

Next you will need to make sure you have placed orders for all your small equipment.

② Ordering Your Small Equipment

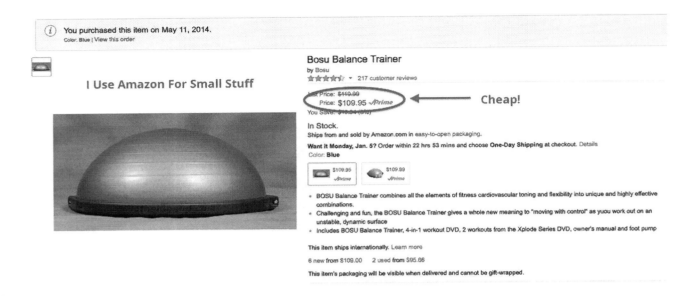

My advice with ordering small equipment is that Amazon is a great resource for deals on up-and-coming fitness brands. In the past I have ordered from the companies below and I will provide links on the resources page of my website.

- Power Systems
- Perform Better
- The Chek Institute
- Iron Company
- Spri
- Palos Sports
- Gopher Sports
- Rogue Fitness
- Muscle Driver

There are many other companies out there and some are fantastic. But I have found that Amazon trumped most of them for small equipment like bosus, bands, balance cushions, foam rollers and more. If you have Amazon Prime, it's even better.

In the resources section of my site, I have posted all my favorite Amazon equipment links, which I used when I opened my last facility. Enjoy them and share any new stuff you find by sending my assistant PJ an email with the name of the equipment and the link to admin@ briandevlin.com. Use the subject line: Resources List Addition.

3 Setting Up Your Online Scheduling & Payment Processing

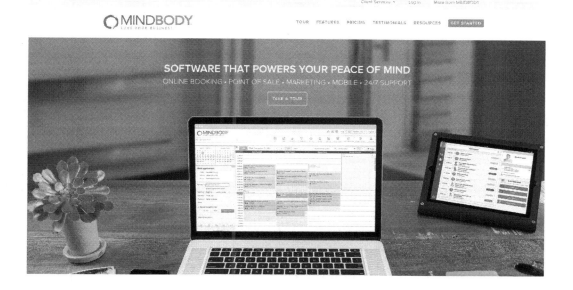

Notice I said "online?" Well, you can learn from my wife, a wonderful woman who refused to give up her day planner or use automated billing for months. After a full year of arguing over more-efficient ways of doing business, she finally decided to admit that online, automated billing and recurring scheduling is the way to go for service-based businesses.

The days of chasing down checks and cash are over for me and I implore you to follow suit. For years, I wasted hours and hours scribbling and erasing check dates and appointment changes in my day planner. In 2006, I finally changed my ways and have not looked back since. In 2008, I bought my first Mac and I have never laid a hand on a PC since that wonderful day. This is how I believe you will feel when you use an automated billing and scheduling system to run your fitness business. Here are my top three recommendations for setting up your online platform. I have personally used two of the three, but a few of my coaching clients use Volo and like it.

1 **Mindbody:** This software is very powerful and gives you so much versatility in performing online scheduling and payment processing. They have the best support department I have seen to date, and you do not have to purchase a third-party payment gateway. Mindbody is a little more expensive than the other two choices, but I think it is worth every penny.

My Bonus! Mindbody is the only software that currently integrates with our FBA platform and I have partnered with them. If you decide to use Mindbody, please sign up for your account using this URL: http://www.FitProEvolution.com/Mindbody/ to receive my FBA 60-day bonus.

Email your receipt to my assistant PJ at admin@briandevlin.com. He will activate a complimentary 60-day FBA account for you so you can test our CRM system with your new business. We will also give you access to our FBA University tutorial videos!

2 **Appointments Plus:** This is reliable online scheduling and payment processing software, but you must use a third-party gateway provider at the same time to handle payments. They also offer limited support, and up-sell you for every add-on. I still use this company in my Charleston location, but we will probably be migrating to Mindbody.

3 **Volo:** I don't have any personal experience with this software, but a few of my high-level coaching clients use this to run their businesses and like it a lot.

Can you still run a successful business without a CRM and a scheduling and payment system? Absolutely! I was booked solid for four years while working out of a North Face backpack and a gym. Will you be stressed, burned out by sending meal plans, cardio programs, surveys, email correspondence and texting? I can honestly say that you may not be. You may be a natural multi-tasker and operate really well with a day planner, cash and checks.

Let me toss in another argument then. What if you are making six-figures, you are popular, respected, booked solid, making a lot of money and one day you get tired of being a trainer or you get hurt? How easy will it be to sell your business to an investor or another trainer if they have no idea how you manage the payments, the scheduling, the value delivery, and on and on? It will be almost impossible. How easy will it be if you want to go in another direction and open a new facility? The bank will ask you for proof of income, a profit-and-loss statement, a copy of your average client load, and want to see proof that you actually have a business.

If you are taking cash and checks and doing what most "shoestring trainers" do — keeping the cash in a safety deposit box, and cashing your checks at your client's banks to avoid making a deposit — you are making two very costly mistakes.

First, you are not going to be paying any taxes, which means you won't show any legitimate income. This means that no lender will take you seriously and you will have a hard time ever growing past your current situation. I know a dozen trainers who operate like this. They hoard their income. They don't invest in growth opportunities or break out of the successful independent contractor mode and into a business mentality.

I knew them 10 years ago and I know them today. Guess what? They are still in the exact same position and making relatively the same income and they will never reach their full potential. Do yourself a favor:

If you are using a day planner and taking checks, invest in one of the above services and start showing legitimate income, efficiency and moving up the totem pole today.

Crafting Your Employee Handbook and SOP

If you are a sole provider right now, you will want to hire employees soon because your lease is a liability and you need to exercise leverage to ensure that you not only break even, but also thrive and grow.

You don't have to start with employees. You can start as a sole provider. But you still need to have a Standard Operating Procedure and an Employee Handbook. It does not have to be a massive document. It might just be a few pages. They can be continuously updated and changed as your business progresses. The purpose of these two documents is to provide two very important elements of leadership and expectations for your staff:

1   Expectation of roles and consequences for behaviors.

2   Guidance and structure for implementing our systems.

I opened a business a few months ago and worked alone for two months until I was 75% booked on Monday, Wednesday and Friday. Once I was 75% booked, I hired my first trainer and put every new lead on her schedule. Once she was 50% booked, I hired my second trainer and split all new leads between her and my first trainer. She is almost 50% booked now and we are interviewing for our third trainer as I write this book. I will continue this process and keep sending traffic to my funnels until we are at 80% max capacity.

At this point, the facility will be generating close to 60K per month in gross revenue and I will have already signed a new lease and be in the fourth week of the new launch process. I know this because it is just a small part of my SOP for hiring new staff. Not only does it give my employees a grander vision, but also allows them to progress as my company progresses.

When I hired my most recent employee, she took great satisfaction in realizing that she could very easily become an owner of her own studio. We would back her 100% in getting it started as long as she worked her way to that level by following our SOP and handbook for advancement.

In the resources section of my website, I offer some tools you can use to create the SOP and handbook you will implement in your dry-run training phase. We also cover this in great detail in my **Fitness Launch Academy** video coaching program, where I provide templates and scripts for almost all the sections of this book.

Next we need to at least start designing our direct-response company website. I will show you how to get a very professional site up and running without breaking the bank.

⑤ Design Your Direct Response Website

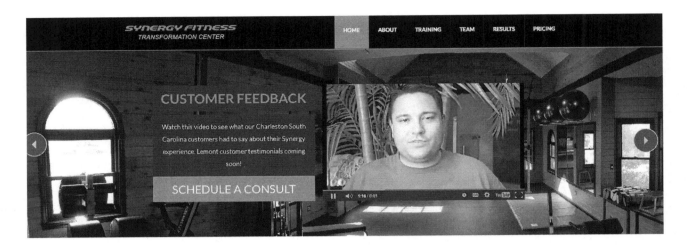

Your website is important. It is one of the first things a potential customer will check out before calling you for a consultation. The website design industry is a very lucrative industry, and most designers get a few thousand dollars to design a business website.

I have good news! You don't have to pay that much. You can actually get a really nice looking site up and running for $500-$1,000 and sometimes even less.

Here is a list of very important elements your direct-response website should have if you want it to steadily attract and convert visitors:

- A compelling headline that speaks to a specific problem customers in your market have
- Features and benefits your customer receives
- A two-step lead magnet delivery system that puts your visitor into an auto responder email sequence
- Social proof like video testimonials and photos showing that you are a reputable provider of services
- An authority graphic showing any major media coverage you have received
- A satisfaction guarantee
- A link to your Facebook fan page

- Pictures of your facility
- Trainer bios and your story
- A consultation request page
- Google map plug-in and contact page showing your address and driving directions
- A specific call to action

 Go to FitProEvolution.com/Resources/ to see the companies I use to find great web site templates for pennies.

 If you would like us to create your website for you through my branding and design company, Idea Inception, please visit our company site at Ideainception.com and submit a request for a design consultation.

We have a full line of branding and identity products from basic website packages to custom platform design.

If you want to do it yourself, follow these seven steps:

1 Go to my resource page and look at our site template partner pages or find your own template.

2 Hire a coder to customize the template to your specifications.

3 Get your stock images purchased and text written.

4 Review your finished design and go through the revision process with your designer.

5 Agree on the final design and pay for the deliverables.

6 Hire the coder to make your site live.

7 Hire an on-page SEO expert to optimize your site for the search engines.

You will probably be online within 30 days, with only a few remaining paid revisions to finalize the site. Otherwise, you should be good to go.

6 **Finding And Hiring Potential Employees**

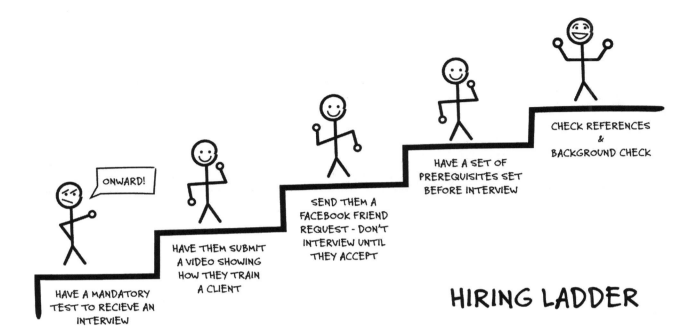

ONWARD!

HAVE A MANDATORY
TEST TO RECIEVE AN
INTERVIEW

HAVE THEM SUBMIT
A VIDEO SHOWING
HOW THEY TRAIN
A CLIENT

SEND THEM A
FACEBOOK FRIEND
REQUEST - DON'T
INTERVIEW UNTIL
THEY ACCEPT

HAVE A SET OF
PREREQUISITES SET
BEFORE INTERVIEW

CHECK REFERENCES
&
BACKGROUND CHECK

HIRING LADDER

Finding and hiring good fitness talent and administration can be a time-consuming task, but I have a few short cuts I use when searching for talent.

1 Ask your friends, family and coworkers if they know of anyone with the skills you are looking for.

2 Use Facebook and post your job requirements on your fan page. Then boost your post and target accordingly.

3 Run a Facebook add to a survey page that has the questions you want answered, and target fitness pros.

4 Purchase the domain name [YourCity]FitnessJobs.com and put up an online application form. Run ads to it.

5 Post your ads on Craigslist (Not my first choice)

6 Post your ads in the help wanted section of your local paper. (Not my favorite either)

How To Interview

I have some resources for good interview questions on my resource page, but here are some things you can do to ensure a higher-quality candidate. Some are extreme, but so is the pain of spending a year developing and training someone who winds up stealing from you or is dishonest.

- Make the applicant jump through some hoops to get an interview.
- Have a mandatory test to receive an interview.
- Make them submit a video showing how they train a client.
- Send the applicant a Facebook friend request and don't interview until they accept.
- Have a specific set of prerequisites that have to be met before the interview.
- Check references before you grant an interview.
- Use Spokeo or a background service agency and run a background check.

The Golden Rule: Hire slow and fire fast. You will usually know within a few weeks if your employee is going to be a perpetual drain on your time, resources and emotional stability. Most bad apples have a history of frequent employment and cannot provide references, but sometimes they will slip under your interview radar and into the ranks of your team.

History repeats itself. If you have one or more instances of "red flag" behavior in the first 30 days, politely dismiss them and wish them well. It will serve you much better long term.

Everything I write in this book is from my 15 years of experience and a collection of bad decisions that I have learned from. I hope that by outlining my mistakes, I can spare you the discomfort of these scenarios occurring in your business.

10 Reasons To Hire

1 The candidate has an unusual energy and enthusiasm that attracts you.

2 The candidate has a history of achievement and holds good references.

3 The candidate understands where you are going, your vision and even offers suggestions.

4 The candidate seems like he/she would be amazing with people.

5 The candidate has confidence, not arrogance.

6 The candidate is on board with your vision, mission, aims and objectives and seems excited.

7 The candidate has actually researched your company.

8 The candidate seems eager to get started.

9 The candidate asks how to help you reach your vision and offers dialogue that corresponds to that.

10 The candidate appears to be highly teachable.

Once you have your final hiring completed, hold a team meeting and let the staff know that they will be entering "dry-run" training in the days to come. Make sure they all understand their roles and expectations. I recommend that you film the meetings so you can use the meeting footage to train management as your business grows. Also make sure that you go over the SOP and employee handbook in detail at your meetings. Employees are only as good as the leadership they receive.

- Lead by example
- Lead with consistency
- Lead with respect and empathy, but don't allow excuses

Always offer your employees a glimpse of the future, and let them feel a sense of ownership and endless advancement opportunities with your company. Never paint the picture that this is all there is. If an employee or any human feels a box around them, they will try to find a way out on their own. If your employee wants to be an owner and sees a grander future for themselves, encourage that. One day they may headline a second or third facility that you can open for them, with the opportunity to buy you out or expand your brand as a partner. Partner with greatness. Don't smother it.

A lot of employees talk big about their future, yet their daily actions don't reflect that dialogue. Entrepreneur is a rare action verb. **Want**repreneur is not. Learn to spot the difference between talk and action in your employees. It will help you realize where you need to apply effort, and where you need to prune dead branches.

My wife commented the other day that "a lot of people are not like you Brian, and you can't hold them accountable to a vision that is too scary for them." I responded by saying, "I didn't scare you did I?"

Be mindful of your vision and make sure you are attracting like-minded employees. They are out there, but she is right. They are a rare breed. When you find one, hold onto them like I do.

138

⑦ Commercial Banking & Merchant Account

This section will be quick. If you have not done this already, you will need to get your commercial banking set up so that you can open your business in a few weeks and accept all major credit cards, checks and cash.

Some states like South Carolina simply require you to have a DBA name and a driver's license; other states like Pennsylvania require you to have your articles of incorporation, proof of lease or home office, and all sorts of identification.

Find out what you need and get that put into your folder and ready to go. I recommend getting the checks that come in a three-ring binder with stubs that remain after you write and tear out a check.

This makes accounting much easier, and can save you the headache of having to log into your online banking and look at each individual check image that you have written.

Here is a quick list of items you may need to get a commercial banking account:

- Driver's license
- Passport
- EIN
- Social Security Card
- Stamped Articles of Incorporation
- Business plan
- Loan approval documentation
- Utility bill for the business
- Copy of your executed lease

It seems like a lot to have, but this is what was required of me in Pennsylvania to start a commercial bank account for my Sub S corporation. I hope you don't have to jump through as many hoops; but if you do, you will be prepared.

Next we need to get insurance on our leased space if we have not already. In the next section, I will review this process and try to save you any headaches

8 — Acquiring Liability Insurance

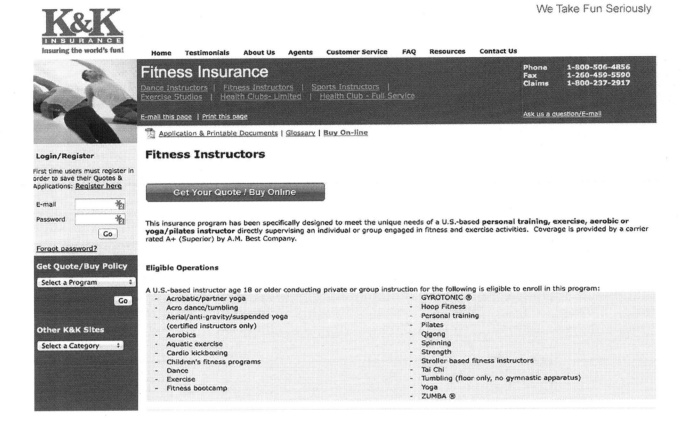

Getting insurance is very easy and can be done online in just a few minutes. Here are some quick things to consider when purchasing insurance:

1 Most commercial leases require $1 million in liability coverage.

2 Most insurance quotes are for you and your facility only. If you have employees or ICs, you will need to either get them insurance or make them carry their own policy. If you go this route, they will need to list your company as "co-insured" or "additionally insured" on the policy, and they will need to bring you proof of that certificate for your company records.

3 If you live in areas prone to natural disaster or flooding, you will most likely not be covered unless it is stated on your policy. Most policies for fitness studios offer this upgrade.

4 Your equipment will not be covered under this policy and you will need to upgrade your policy to cover personal property up to a specified amount. This can drastically increase the overall cost of your policy, so make sure you understand what you are being charged for, and that you have an itemized list of your covered items.

5 You may be asked if you want sexual harassment or emergency medical coverage for your employees added to your policy. This will be a decision you have to make as well.

Once you have your policy, you should receive an email if it was an online transaction. If it was a local offline transaction, you will have hard copies. Give a copy of your insurance to your landlord if they request it.

That's about all I have ever had to decide when buying my insurance policies. I hope the process goes smoothly for you too, and that neither of us ever have to use our benefits.

 I have listed some insurance companies I use in the resources section of my website at FitProEvolution.com/Resources/

Next, we will need to make sure all our employee, contractor and customer paperwork is created. We will cover this in the next section.

⑨ Drawing Up Your Legal Paperwork

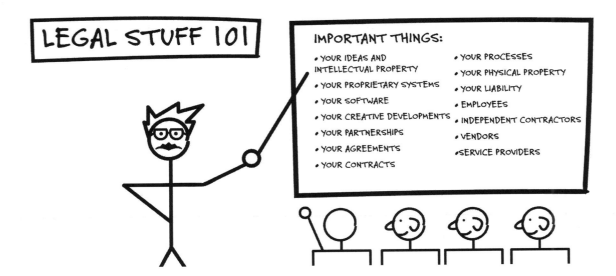

LEGAL STUFF 101

IMPORTANT THINGS:
- YOUR IDEAS AND INTELLECTUAL PROPERTY
- YOUR PROPRIETARY SYSTEMS
- YOUR SOFTWARE
- YOUR CREATIVE DEVELOPMENTS
- YOUR PARTNERSHIPS
- YOUR AGREEMENTS
- YOUR CONTRACTS
- YOUR PROCESSES
- YOUR PHYSICAL PROPERTY
- YOUR LIABILITY
- EMPLOYEES
- INDEPENDENT CONTRACTORS
- VENDORS
- SERVICE PROVIDERS

When drawing up legal paperwork, always grab a standard copy of something online at my favorite legal site, (on my resources page) and then I pay my attorney a nominal fee to alter it slightly if need be so that I am fully protected while I do business. Below is a list of items you want to build expectation and protection around with your legal agreements:

- Your ideas and intellectual property
- Your proprietary systems
- Your software
- Your creative developments
- Your partnerships
- Your agreements
- Your contracts
- Your processes
- Your physical property
- Your liability
- Employees
- Independent contractors
- Vendors
- Service providers

I give access to all my forms, agreement templates and company process maps to members of my **Fitness Launch Academy Coaching Program**. This will save you thousands in legal fees.

 You can get instant access at FitnessLaunchAcademy.com.

The only action items left are passing our final inspections, setting up our payroll systems and reviewing the list to make sure we are on track. Next we will move into our "dry-run" training phase where we pull a targeted number of test-clients into our funnel and take them through our entire process.

CHAPTER NINE

Dry-Run Training

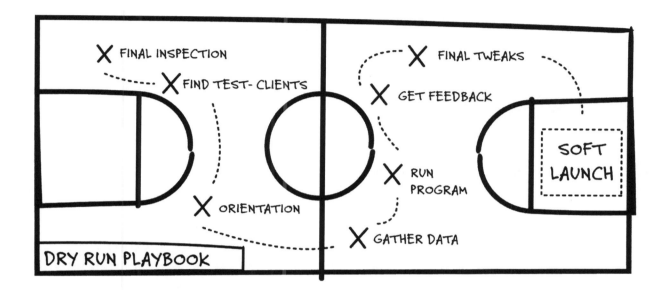

In dry-run training, our primary objective is to break our system. When software developers release new software, they usually go through a phase called beta testing. During this time, their only objective is to see if they can play the role of an inexperienced user and do five things:

- Find weak links and unprotected areas
- Find a way to cause an error message or crash the software
- Find dead ends and unsupported processes
- Obtain user experience feedback
- Review analytic data and watch user trends

Then they take all that feedback and repair the software before releasing it to the public.

Think of yourself during this week as a software tester for your fitness software. It is your job to find out where you are failing your customers, employees and business. Then you need to repair those weak areas to make your brand bulletproof, attractive and one your clients can connect with easily.

The format of these last three chapters will not be broken down into days. They will be presented as a series of steps, some extremely obvious and others maybe giving you an 'aha' moment.

My only goal is to have you prepared, informed and ready to face any obstacle that threatens your facility opening — and your confidence.

You can do this! It's going to be life-changing and you are going to be very successful. Just stay the course and don't ever give up.

OK, let's go over your final inspection items and beta test your venture so we can push your business with confidence through this final launch sequence.

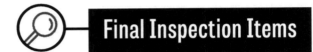

Final Inspection Items

1 Is your certificate of occupancy posted?

       Yes   No

It's a good idea to frame and post your business license and certificate of occupancy on the wall in your reception area or where you get the most traffic from walk-ins. Often, after a business has passed its certification, building inspectors will come and check that you have your documentation visible. Especially if there was a previous altercation.

2 Are your fire suppression systems inspected and labeled well?

       Yes   No

Your local fire inspector will usually give you a fire suppression certificate that is good for one year. Fold this up and put it in a plastic bag and zip tie it to the fire extinguisher hanger. That way it will always be right there and you will never scramble when they come to inspect.

3 Are your exits clearly labeled?

       Yes   No

This can hold up your final inspection and can always leave you open for a lawsuit if someone were trapped in your building for any reason. Just make sure you have exit signs up. They are inexpensive and will save you headaches with the code office and lawyers.

4 Do you have obvious customer traffic pattern set up?

Yes   No

This is an optional item, but when surveying customers of my first establishment, I found that they felt there was a big traffic bottleneck by the front desk because clients left and entered via a small hallway formed by the coat area and front desk. We had two doors, so we put the dirty towel hamper by the second door and the new towel bin by the first door. This caused an involuntary shift in the traffic patterns and my reviews went up.

5 Are your water fountains functioning well?

Yes   No

You'll get big complaints when water fountains are warm or taste bad. I have received two requests for spring water coolers in my South Carolina location. People like their water fountains cold, crisp and clean. Keep them that way!

6 Are your floors installed and clean?

Yes   No

Walk your floor and make sure that there are no bubbles in the rubber or splintered areas if they are wood. If they are cement, make sure they are not slippery and that they are clean.

7 Are all the painting supplies removed?

Yes   No

Construction materials tend to sit around for months after a new gym is opened. They are usually in a cabinet or a closet, or in some cases in a corner. Make sure you remove all construction material. Customers notice this stuff more than you think.

8 Is there any blue painter's tape on the walls?

Yes   No

Same concept. Make sure you do a walk-through and grab all the tape remnants if you painted.

9   Are all the light bulbs working?

Yes   No

Customers notice when light bulbs are out. I recommend that you add a daily bulb check to your manager's SOP when you reach that stage. I have had surveys come back with simple stuff like this being known to aggravate customers.

10   Are all the outlet covers back on and paint free?

Yes   No

This is another insidious little customer grievance item. After you paint a facility or do work, make sure you replace all the electrical outlet and light switch covers and remove any paint that may have spilled on them.

11   Are all the minor construction holes patched and painted?

Yes   No

Just like light switches and outlet covers, there always seem to be areas where the drywall has not been sanded and painted. Fix this before your soft launch.

12   Is the sound system hooked up?

Yes   No

I had to run out to Guitar Center 24 hours before my second studio opened to buy a PA system for my studio. I had forgotten the sound system. Make sure yours is working and you have a few backups. Keep an old MP3 player around if you are using the internet to feed your sound system. At my second studio location, we used Pandora. When the internet went out one day, we had to scramble and get one of the trainers to bring their iPod in to plug into the PA system. Make sure you have a few backup devices for your sound system. Sound is very important in a fitness center.

13   Is your internet hooked up?

Yes   No

In all the chaos of opening your facility, don't forget to turn your internet on. Also make sure that you get at least a week or two of lead time, because companies like Comcast and Time Warner can be booked up for weeks. It would not be good if your opening was held up because you simply did not have internet and could not process payments.

14 Is your plumbing operational and do you have water?

Yes   No

In order to get your certificate of occupancy, your plumbing needs to be operational. Sometimes, your landlord may be paying your water bill while you're building out your space. Make sure the water bill has been transferred into your name prior to opening. It would be quite a disappointment if your opening was held up because you couldn't flush the toilets.

15 Is your dumpster set up?

Yes   No

In opening my third facility, I made the mistake of forgetting to pay the dumpster fee. When you order large pieces of equipment, they come with a bunch of shrink wrap, metal wire, pallets, and cardboard. I had to personally rent a truck and haul this trash to the dump, which was physically taxing and expensive. Don't forget to pay your dumpster fee.

16 Is your sign installed?

Yes   No

Although this is not mandatory for opening, and many businesses open before signage is up, I do recommend having your sign installed and visible prior to your opening. This will help attract your target market during your launch phase. It is the easiest form of passive marketing that you otherwise will miss out on.

17 Have you changed the locks?

Yes   No

Don't make the mistake of putting $30,000-$50,000 of new equipment in your facility and then forgetting to change the locks. You have no idea who had keys to your facility before you rented it and most landlords do not change locks between tenants unless it's specified in the lease.

18 Is your security system working?

Yes   No

You may or may not have a security system installed in your new facility. If you do, and you wish to use an alarm system, make sure that your account is current before filling your space with expensive items. The need for a security system will vary from town to town, but it's always a good thing to have.

19 Are your fire alarms working?

Yes   No

Prior to opening, test all of your installed smoke detectors manually. Replace any dead batteries and make sure all fire extinguishers are up to date.

20 Is your equipment set up and operational?

Yes   No

Make sure that you have assembled, inspected, and tested all of your equipment prior to taking test clients. I made the mistake of not inspecting my new cable cross-over from Iron Company until I was training clients with it. While doing cable chest flies, the weight stack actually got stuck because one of the guide rods was slightly warped. It was embarrassing for me, and potentially hazardous for my client. Since I waited more than two weeks after my equipment was delivered before reporting the problem, my warranty was voided and Iron Company was of no help. Don't let this happen to you; inspect every piece of equipment before use!

21 Is the equipment clean?

Yes   No

New does not equal clean. Equipment sits in warehouses for months before it is shipped and delivered. Most equipment comes with a layer of cardboard dust and sometimes oil on the surface. Wipe down all dumbbells and remove any excess shipping oil, and wipe down all upholstery and metal on your equipment prior to opening. You never get a second chance at a first impression.

22 Is the equipment stored neatly on the wall or is it sitting on the floor?

Yes   No

This is my biggest pet peeve. If you know me, there is a hook, hanger, or some device to secure any and all pieces of equipment in my facilities to the wall or off the floor. From sand bags and bands, to kettle bells and medicine balls, nothing sits on my floor. Visual clutter can ruin your customer experience.

23 Are your bathrooms in working order, stocked and clean?

Yes   No

I recommend stocking your bathroom with large toilet paper rolls and automatic paper towel dispensers, as well as soap dispensers on the wall, hand sanitizers and air fresheners. While surveying my clients, I found many times these items were requested, so they are now standard in each facility. We also keep a container of feminine products in the bathroom as well.

24 Is your front desk or reception area set up?

Yes   No

Make sure your front desk is clean, free of clutter, and contains your check-in system, company brochures, and gift cards. I find that customers often take brochures and gift cards for friends and family when they check out.

25 Is there adequate storage for customer belongings?

Yes   No

I recommend a bin or locker system near the front check-in area for customers to store personal items, such as purses, wallets, keys, cell phones, and personal effects. Customers that I surveyed prefer to have a private area to store these things.

26 Are there adequate coat hangers or hooks?

Yes   No

If your facility is in a warm climate, this may not be as much of a factor to consider. But my newest facility is in Pennsylvania and the winters are quite cold. We need adequate storage and hooks for hanging 12-20 jackets. We also need storage for winter boots, gloves and hats, etc. Keep climate in mind when designing your facility.

27 Is your payment processor set up?

Yes   No

This is probably the most important item on this checklist. Without money coming in on a recurring basis, you have no predictable income. Make sure your payment processor is hooked up and all gateways are functional before taking on test clients. I recommend running a payment with your own card and observing the process before taking any customer payments.

28 Is your scheduling system set up?

Yes   No

Digital scheduling is paramount to your success, because most scheduling services are hosted on secure servers with redundant backup systems. Your day planner could be lost or stolen in the blink of an eye. Do not open your facility without a reputable online appointment scheduling system in place. I have recommended three in previous chapters of this book.

29 Is your paperwork printed?

Yes   No

I recommend printing out multiple copies of all your paperwork and placing them in organization bins on the wall in your consultation and check-in areas. This way you can quickly see if you are getting low on copies and it keeps the whole paperwork process very organized and helps avoid visual clutter of papers stacked on desks.

30 Is your check-in area organized?

Yes   No

Double-check your client check-in area and ask yourself this question: "If I were a client of this facility, how would I feel about approaching this desk?" If you feel good, chances are so will your future clients.

31 Are your brochures on display?

Yes   No

I recommend placing your brochures in a display container that sits vertically in your check-in area, as opposed to setting them on a counter. Your clients will be more likely to notice them and possibly grab some to distribute on your behalf.

32 Are your gift cards on display?

       Yes   No

Gift cards are better than business cards in my opinion. I discussed this in a previous chapter. I recommend having your gift cards on display for prospects and customers to grab. Even if your gift is nothing more than a free consultation valued at $67, it will foster reciprocity on the part of your clients and prospects.

33 Are your pricing sheets printed?

       Yes   No

Customers really appreciate being able to see pricing in writing. Use pricing sheets during consultations, so that your prospect knows that everyone receives the same price for your services. Make sure your pricing sheets correspond to your company website, if applicable.

34 Do you have a first aid kit?

       Yes   No

One of my trainers got their finger cut on a snap hook while using the dual cable machine with a client. When she ran over and asked me for a Band-Aid, I regretfully remembered that the first aid kit I had ordered was still at my house. The customer had to run out to her car to grab a Band-Aid for my employee. This is why I will always have a first aid kit under the desk.

35 Is your personal office set up?

       Yes   No

Your personal office is a very important part of your business. It is where you brainstorm, strategize, and take care of business. Make sure that your office is a place where you don't mind spending time. If you don't have an office, you can always use a local coffee shop or some inspirational venue to get away from the grind and do the mind work necessary to move your business forward.

36 Do you have a computer?

Yes   No

If you don't, you need to get one. I recommend Mac. You can usually pick up an older 21-inch iMac in great condition on Craigslist for a few hundred dollars. Your customers will look at you like you have three heads if you don't check them in and out on some sort of reliable electronic scheduling system.

37 Do you have a printer?

Yes   No

You can find these for pennies on Craigslist, but I recommend having one at the check-in area for printing receipts.

38 Are your office supplies stocked?

Yes   No

Nothing is worse than running out of printer paper while you're printing an important document. Make sure all of your office supplies are stocked and that you have an inventory system for staples, paper clips, copy paper, tape, pens, and all the necessary office equipment you will use on regular basis.

39 Do you have a white board?

Yes   No

I love white boards. I use white boards constantly. They help me drill down into what it is I really need to accomplish every week and help me map out complicated business ideas. If you don't have a whiteboard you should get one.

40 Do you have ample post it notes?

Yes   No

This is my secret weapon. Post it notes are amazing for mapping out processes, because you can put the title of one of your processes on each note and move them around on your wall until you see a system or an idea that works perfectly. I am a big visual learner and mapper, so this might not be something that you're interested in. But you can always use them for taking messages.

41   Are your legal docs set up?

       Yes   No

This is super important: Don't train anyone without proper legal documentation, such as health histories, PAR-Q's, waivers, and informed consent forms. Cover your bases legally.

42   Is your programming laid out?

       Yes   No

We use three-ring binders with our classes and periodized programs, all mapped out and ready to be added to our trainer's itinerary. I recommend you implement some sort of repeatable and teachable program design model in your facility.

43   Is your SOP printed and ready for distribution?

       Yes   No

Make sure your SOP and employee handbook are finished prior to your first team meeting. It is very important that you give your employees a strong framework from which to operate, grow, and thrive.

44   Do you have at least one sales funnel fully set up?

       Yes   No

Before your soft opening, you should have your first sales funnel completely set up and automated, whether the traffic comes from online or offline sources. For more information on this topic, see chapter 5.

45   Is your conversion process dialed in and locked down?

       Yes   No

Remember, you will only be as successful as your conversion process. Does your prospect consistently take your lead magnet and follow it all the way to your core offering? Make sure this is dialed in before you open the doors.

46 Have you role-played the process with employees?

Yes   No

This is important. During your team meeting, have your staff role play consultations with each other, and make sure they understand and can implement your conversion system efficiently and effectively. Try using difficult scenarios so that your team understands how to overcome objections to the sale.

47 Are you ready to hold orientation?

Yes   No

Orientation is when you take your test clients through your entire conversion system, all the way to your core offering, and treat them just as if you were already open. Look for weak links in your system and obtain feedback from your test clients through detailed surveys and personal interviews.

48 Are you ready to train test-subjects?

Yes   No

Only you can answer this. If you've answered yes to most of the questions on this list, you're probably in pretty good shape. Trust your instincts, and trust your gut feelings.

49 Is your team ready to rock?

Yes   No

Does your team seem excited? Maybe it's just you. Don't worry, you will have a team soon. If you do have employees, now is the time to take an honest look at who comprises your dream team and decide whether or not they truly fit the culture you've worked so hard to design. If you need to make adjustments at this point, do it quickly and decisively.

50 Are you ready to do this?

Yes   No

Of course you are! You've waited your whole life for this. You can't fail. There is no plan B. This is do-or-die. I believe in you, you believe in you and the world is going to be a better place with your fitness business thriving in it. Let's do this.

Finding Test Clients For Your Fat Loss Study Or Dry-Run Training

Note: You don't have to use a fat loss study, but if you use the word study it already implies that you will be gathering objective and subjective data. You are much less likely to run into compliance issues if you phrase it as a study. Studies carry more authority and respect than the word "promo" as well.

There are literally hundreds of ways to generate interest in becoming a test client of your facility. You can easily do this by making a list of 50 friends, family members and acquaintances. Then reach out to these people and offer them a completely free or heavily discounted experience. But remember, they must adhere to certain stipulations that I have listed below.

1 They must be willing to be photographed and measured before they start training.

This is important and you will need to have them sign a film and video release before taking any pictures of them. I recommend you do this in a large orientation group where you will go over all your expectations and rules for being part of your fat loss study.

2 They must be willing to be filmed for video and give video feedback about their experience.

You are doing this to gather testimonials and social proof that your programming and business model work for most people. Make sure that your test subjects understand that this part is required and not optional.

3 They must be present for at least 85% of the sessions offered.

Attendance issues will ruin your results. If you want to attract your target market after your facility is open to the public, then you will need to choose good test subjects now who have the freedom to make the sessions without incident. For instance, you would not want to choose a single mother with three children and no other source of childcare to be a test subject, because she will most likely run into dozens of issues when it comes to adhering to your requirements, simply because she can't help the setbacks that are likely to ensue with her lack of support. This may sound cold, but after you are successfully opened, you will have time to give back to the community. Put on your own oxygen mask first so you can help others later by choosing the right test subject in advance.

4   They must be willing to fill out before, during and after surveys about their experience.

Honest feedback is the only way you can remove blind spots in your business. Make sure your test subjects know that they need to report on the good, the bad, and the ugly in order for you to improve the experience for all involved.

5   They must be in a position where they really want to change.

The last thing you want is test subjects who are just doing this because it sounds fun. Your test subjects need to be extremely frustrated with their health in order to truly embrace this chance for change. Do not hire a bunch of bubbly cute girls that photograph well to be your test subjects, unless you want your fat loss study to be a total joke.

6   They must be easy to work with and follow instructions without arguing.

No Negative Nancy's and Ned's! Only accept people who are positive, want real change and believe you are the one to help them get it. Negative people will bring the entire energy of the experiment to a screeching halt, and they also may resist giving credit where credit is due when testimonial time rolls around.

7   They must not have any physical limitations that would keep them from completing your program.

Again, you will have plenty of time to give back to the community and I implore you to do so after you are up and running. Your beta testing time is not the best time to work with special populations unless that is ultimately your target market. I'm not trying to sound cold, just suggesting that even community service needs to be strategically developed in order to be effective.

8   They must be willing to post on social media daily.

They must be willing to post a progress picture and picture of a meal they are eating to their Facebook timeline every day. They also need to say a few words about their experience that day, and something they learned about themselves. They also need to tag your Fan Page and you as the trainer.

Hold Your Orientation

This does not have to be fancy and can be as simple as 12-20 chairs in your studio and a whiteboard, or even a Google hangout. It can also be ornate and huge. It is completely up to you and your individual situation.

You may be a one-person show right now and that is completely fine! You only need 5-10 people to make this work like gangbusters. Just five people going through this fat loss study will yield:

- 5 sets of before-and-after photos
- 5 written testimonials
- 5 video testimonials
- 5 new perspectives on your business and how to make it better
- 5 Facebook case studies
- 1 documentary video for release
- Dozens of pictures for your website
- Tons of word of mouth advertising
- Tons of Facebook advertising
- Much more

The Ten Step "Grand Slam" Orientation Process

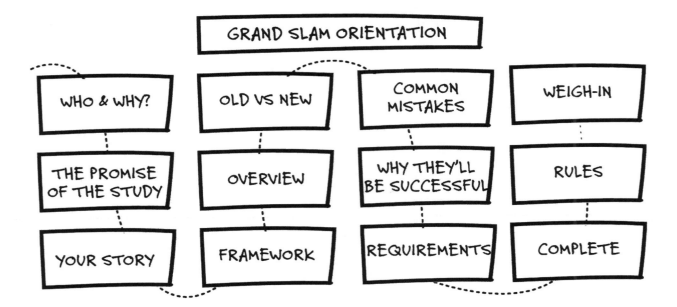

Be sure to cover the following topics/action steps in order for the best engagement and conversion:

- Who you are and your big "why" for doing what you do
- The promise of the study and what it will do for them
- Your story of struggle and your story of finding the truth
- The old way of doing things (vs) the new way
- Overview of your new framework & why your way is special
- The actual framework piece-by-piece
- Where people make mistakes and what they should be aware of when using your system
- Why they are going to be successful with your program
- What you need from them and what you won't tolerate
- Complete all the weigh-ins, pictures, before videos, measurements
- Give them their action sheets

End your orientation class by pumping them up about the results they are going to experience over the next 14-30 days. Give them their daily requirements sheet to take with them. Give them gift cards and flyers to hand out to their friends, family and co-workers. Let them know that you can't succeed without their help, support and adherence to your program.

You have now established a loyal tribe, and if you did your job in the orientation process, they will follow you to the ends of the earth. They know you, they trust you, and they like you. Don't let them down. Make this their best experience ever. Pour into them and give them every ounce of your encouragement, devotion and belief. It will serve you and it will serve them. Leaders give. They bleed and fight alongside their platoons. Be a leader!

Note: This process is involved and time-consuming but well worth it. I have compiled everything you need to run your fat loss study successfully, and made it available to members of the **Fitness Launch Academy** coaching program.

 You can learn more about becoming a member at FitnessLaunchAcademy.com.

Your Applied Test Client Process

I am not going to coach you on this. You are opening a fitness business because you believe you have a powerful gift that the world needs. For me to tell you how to use that gift would not be appropriate. I will offer some advice about the outcomes though.

- Make sure that your classes are organized
- Make sure that you touch and call everyone by name during each class
- Catch them doing things right and be careful when critically analyzing their actions
- Make the process easy to follow. Step-by-step instructions and expectations are important
- Give them your all
- Follow up daily using a private Facebook group
- Give them all the tools they need to succeed
- Hold them accountable to their end. If they don't follow instructions, gently call them out
- Make it fun
- Make it memorable
- Give them your gear to wear if you have it
- Above all, make it work!

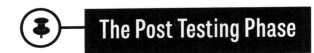

The Post Testing Phase

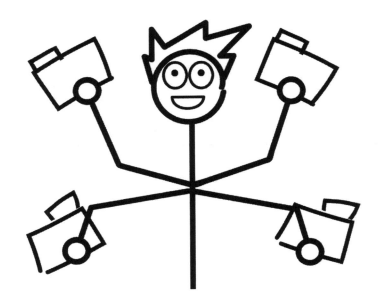

- CREATE A MARKETING FOLDER
  - COMPANY LOGO
  - COMPANY VIDEO
  - SUB FOLDERS FOR EACH TEST CLIENT
  - SCREENSHOTS FROM YOUR FACEBOOK GROUP
  - GROUP PHOTOS

- REVIEW YOUR THREE SURVEYS
  - BEFORE
  - DURING
  - AFTER

- MAKE ANY NECESSARY CHANGES
  - LOOK AT YOUR SURVERYS
  - MAKE ANY CHANGES OR CORRECTIONS

You will have so much data after this process, if you complete it the right way. You will have dozens of progress photos and Facebook posts you can screenshot. You will have individual video testimonials from each person involved. You will have hundreds of action photos. You will have an awesome group photo for your website and much, much more.

If you follow the dry-run training protocols set down in this book or my **Fitness Launch Academy Program**, you will have everything you need to solidify your brand and your new position as a local authority on fat loss or whatever your brand signifies.

Here is a list of vital action steps you should implement after you complete your dry run promo:

√ ── Create a marketing folder on your computer with the following items in it:

1 Your company logo

2 Your company video intro stinger

3 A sub folder for each test client containing:

- Screenshots of all their Facebook posts during the study
- Copies of their daily journal
- Copies of all their action photos
- Copies of their before and graduation photo
- Copy of their video testimonial
- Copy of their before and after stats
- Copies of their daily progress shots
- Test subject bio

4 Screenshots from your Facebook group

5 Group photos

✓ —— Review your three surveys

Before survey: The questions you asked them before they started.

During Survey: The questions you asked them while they were in the study.

After Survey: The questions you ask them after the study was completed.

✓ —— Make the necessary changes needed and correct the deficiencies discovered by your fat loss study.

- Look at your before surveys and tweak your attraction process
- Look at your during surveys and tweak your class or training structure, staff, activities, and SOP
- Look at your after surveys and tweak your processes, communication, the whole nine yards

That's it! You are ready to launch your business to the public. You have strategically created a bulletproof offering and you have wowed the members of your test study.

Don't overthink this. You just have to repeat what you just did on a larger scale now.

You don't have to go out and rent a hotel ballroom or go on live TV. You just have to increase the numbers to your comfort level. You have just over-delivered to 5-10 members of your target market, so if you set up your pricing right, by retaining these members in your program, you will most likely be at break-even levels or better.

Just do it again for your soft launch, but set your sights a little higher by strategically locating and attracting your target market.

If you are confused at this point it's OK. This is a simple, yet complex process. If it were super easy, everyone would be doing it and you would have much more competition. Chances are, if you follow the principles and strategies outlined in this book, you will quickly rise to the top of your market, even if it is dominated by veterans. The information provided in this book is not readily available and you have a distinct advantage over your competition because you have this information and they probably don't.

I have broken down this entire process into easy-to-follow videos and downloadable templates you can use to speed up the implementation.

 You can learn more about my video coaching program and trainer community by visiting FitnessLaunchAcademy.com.

There is no question in my mind that anyone could take the information presented in this book and successfully launch or re-launch an existing fitness business to take it to the next level. But the **Fitness Launch Academy** will remove any and all guesswork associated with implementing the strategies and tactics presented in this book.

CHAPTER TEN

Your Soft Launch

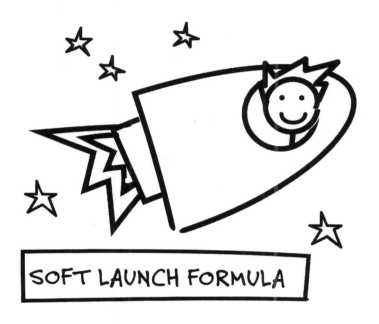

SOFT LAUNCH FORMULA

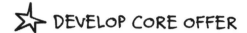 DEVELOP CORE OFFER

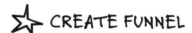 CREATE FUNNEL

RUN PROGRAM

MEASURE CONVERSIONS ACROSS STAGES

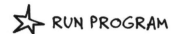 GATHER FEEDBACK & DATA

TWEAK SCALE - REPEAT

I'll be completely transparent here. You may be done if you successfully execute the steps outlined in this chapter. I personally have never had the need or desire for a grand opening because my soft launches usually put me in the green and allowed me to slowly and consistently build my brands to the $3 million mark and beyond.

I have included a chapter in this book covering the grand opening steps in detail. But honestly, if you nail the dry run and soft launch you will probably never need to do a grand opening.

So let's dive into the soft launch process and get your business generating real income and freedom for you.

You will need all the objective data you gathered from your dry run training, so hopefully you have it all in the folder I instructed you to create, or at least somewhere you can access easily. This is your launch swipe file. It is what will give you instant credibility and influence with your market.

What we are going to do is make a select target market (3-4 times the size of your break-even member numbers) a very unique offer. We are going to drop these hot, warm and cold leads into the funnel you have designed.

I will outline the exact soft-launch process we used for my latest studio in Pennsylvania so you can conceptually see exactly how it worked. I have even made the ad copy, ad targeting parameters, social media strategy and initial presentation PDF available to members of my "area exclusive" **Fitness Launch Academy** program.

 You can learn more about this program by visiting FitnessLaunchAcademy.com.

OK, let's dive into soft-launch science. A soft launch is a very strategic event that a business owner will use to incrementally build their member numbers by over-delivering to a select target market in a controlled environment and then using this experience to do two things:

- Build a customer base that will stay for life
- Build a massive social proof arsenal that will fuel your next soft launch

Some business owners stop here and just use a perpetual soft-launch formula. They only take customers every 6-8 weeks and an interested prospect will have to wait for the next orientation.

I have seen fellow business owners have great success with this perpetual launch model, with each new launch consistently more involved than the next. It works! It's just not my style. It may appeal to you and if it does, just tweak and repeat the activities of your first launch and expand your target.

① A Funnel Is A Funnel Is A Funnel

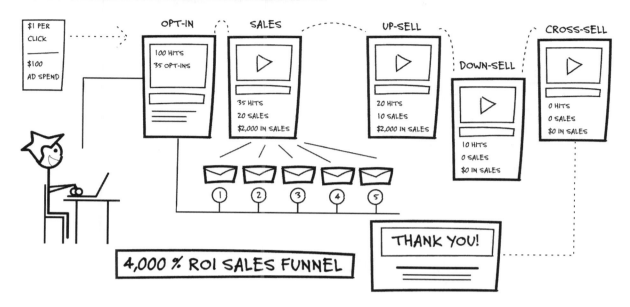

Once you have established a funnel that works, the next step is to scale that funnel to fit your desired work flow and income goals.

A little known fact that 90% of fitness professionals don't understand: Growing a business is simply a matter of knowing your conversion rates at each stage of your funnel. See below for an easy to understand example of a funnel you can use.

- ✓ — 100 people hit your squeeze page; 35 people get your lead magnet.

- ✓ — Those 35 people are redirected to your tripwire offer; 20 people take your offer.

- ✓ — Those 20 people are taken to your core offer and 10 take it.

- $ — You just made 10 new customers and your sales funnel has a 10% total conversion rate.

That means for every 100 people that land on your squeeze page (or ad containing access to your lead magnet), 10 will follow the process all the way through to becoming your customer. The monthly value of a customer is between $97 and $600 per month right now in fitness, depending on the tier or program they fall into.

Let's do the math. What would you be willing to pay per month in advertising to add between $970 and $6,000 to your monthly bottom line? What if it cost you between $1 and $2 to get a lead to land on your squeeze page or print ad? For $200 per month in strategically targeted advertising, you will typically yield somewhere between $970 and $6,000. So now that you know you have a positive ROI on your funnel, you can scale it to whatever size you are comfortable with.

Here is something that you may not have thought about as well:

- Each stage in your funnel can be tweaked if you know the conversion rate. Let's look at the above example.
- Your lead magnet has a 35% conversion rate with cold traffic.
- Your tripwire has a 57% conversion rate with warm traffic (warm because they liked your lead magnet).
- Your core offer has a 50% conversion rate with warm traffic (warm because they liked your tripwire).

What would happen if we only got a 10% conversion rate on our lead magnet and everything else stayed the same?

- For every 100 visitors to our lead magnet, 10 would take it.
- Of those 10 people, roughly 6 would take your tripwire offer.
- Of those 6 people, roughly 3 would take your core offer.

Now our projected monthly income addition would be $291 - $1,800, and our total funnel conversion rate would drop to 3%. This is why you not only need a lead magnet offer that converts, you also need to make sure every stage of your funnel converts. Spend time making sure that the stages of your funnel adhere to all the parameters discussed in Chapter 5. If you don't have a funnel that works, your soft launch won't be as successful as you had hoped.

Unfortunately, most fitness pros think that their good name and superior skill will take them to the top. This is why they struggle to make 50K while the real players sit back and figure out their conversion metrics. Starbucks is a perfect example of this. I have looked into the Starbucks franchise model and they will not open a Starbucks without carefully surveying the demographics. They know their conversion rates at every stage of their funnel from the drive-through images and the way the barista speaks with you, to the sounds you are guaranteed to hear while inside the cafe. They know their numbers and know that they need a certain viable number of their market demographic to land on their lead magnet, which may be nothing more than seeing their sign on the road. Starbucks is not using hope marketing. They are using an equation they can repeat over and over with consistent conversion numbers at every stage of the funnel.

Now that you understand the importance of strategic algebraic marketing, I will outline our latest soft launch activities and show you how easy it is to create a funnel that converts like gangbusters and gives you stability. I am not afraid to take a vacation. I know that while I am gone I can drive traffic to my funnels and my systems will do the rest. As long as all my employees don't call in sick on the same day, we are fortified from lead magnet opt-ins to daily operations, and we have only had this location open about three months.

I Knew Nobody!

I want you to understand that when I opened my most recent location, I knew nobody. We had just left Charleston the year before and moved to Pennsylvania so we could finally experience four seasons again. Yes, I love winter! Well, I decided to take time off while my other facility paid the bills and do something I have always wanted to do. I decided to start a software company. I also decided to use the same exact launch formula outlined here to help my wife open her chiropractic office from scratch in a town where we knew absolutely nobody.

With the exception of a few hiccups, both ventures went off without a hitch. My wife used our launch methods to get more than 100 patients in the first year and has since added another 100. My software company, **Fitness Business Assistant**, was a little slower to take off because we had some problems with the initial platform. But we have since had a massive influx of new trainers and fitness pros, and even chiropractors, using it to greatly simplify their lives. I am proud to say we have more than 100 fitness pros using FBA to simplify their life and we have not even done a full-scale launch or used any advertising!

Shortly after we started the process of creating our new businesses, my wife, Kim, realized that we were pregnant and would soon be parents. Although this was the most amazing news, it also changed the game for good and made me realize that I had to be 10 times more strategic from this point forward.

If you are a parent you understand that children are all-consuming and require every second of your attention when they are babies. Yes, it is wonderful, but let's be honest: If you don't have your game together with your business, a child will sabotage an entrepreneur's ability to get work done, especially from home.

I love my daughter, Charli, with all my heart and I will do whatever it takes to give her an amazing life so that she does not have to face the same struggles I faced growing up. So I wrapped up the development of my software company and outsourced the upkeep so members would be extremely happy. I then set out to open a new facility right here in the town where I spent 22 years of my young adult life. What I am about to outline is exactly how I got this venture off the ground and profitable within a few months — and how you can too. The process I used to open my newest facility is the exact process I have outlined in this book. You now hold the right to (ethically) steal my entire process and, hopefully, have the same level of success or more.

② The Soft-Launch Strategy

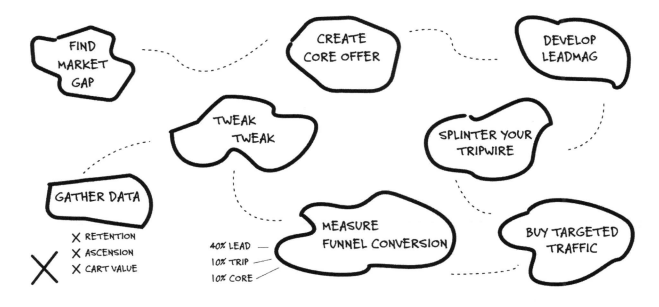

In a town where I know nobody, I was truly challenged in my belief that I could actually make this happen with the same level of success that I had with my previous facilities. I was determined to make this happen, though, and I studied the masters in funnel conversion. I went back into my psychology books and looked for a way that I could set the hook in a town full of strangers.

I looked at all the offerings and tested most of them out to see how I felt as a customer. I even tried to partner with a local guy, but realized there might be too many logistical sticking points to move forward. I had to find the hook. I had to find some way that I could come in and make a huge new statement. Having recently read the book, "Thinkertoys," I became acquainted with the acronym, S.C.A.M.P.E.R, which explained how to take an idea that is already working and make it even better.

- **S**ubstitute
- **C**ombine
- **A**dapt
- **M**odify
- **P**ut to another use
- **E**liminate
- **R**everse

There were a ton of group fitness places in my area. There was one very popular personal training facility and there were a few gyms.

I noticed a gap in the market. There were no small group training facilities that had decent equipment, or facilities that guaranteed body transformations. Nobody really used direct-response advertising and nobody was posting social proof. All websites and offerings were good, but vanilla.

There was one yoga and personal training facility that really understood branding and had really honed in on the stay-at-home mom who was already fit and attractive.

So I decided to adapt small group and private training to a specific market of infrequent exercisers, people who suffered from a slow metabolism (and wanted to improve it), and folks who were self-conscious about being in large groups.

I created my lead magnet and tripwires to attract deconditioned women who were feeling bad about themselves and really desired change. I really enjoy working with individuals who are actually thankful for the help you provide.

I soon realized that I had hit a great market to work with. I absolutely love my clients. Some who were not fit and not happy with their life are already getting dozens of comments and compliments from friends, family and coworkers.

Referrals shortly follow compliments. I get emails almost daily from customers and subscribers around the world thanking me for investing in their life and crossing their path. This feeling cannot be bought and it is wonderful to know you are truly helping where the market failed to show up. It is even better knowing that you can feed your family by helping others in this way.

One of the most common questions I get asked is: "How do you find time to run businesses, have a family, enjoy life and grow every year, while still staying healthy and active?"

The short answer is automation, and the long answer is creating funnels that solve problems, draw people in and create powerful reciprocal relationships for life.

Let's go back to my soft-launch process. I knew I wanted to reach women who were struggling with self-image issues, health, metabolism, energy loss and time constraints. So I had a specific idea for a funnel that would work well.

I also recognized that, as a newcomer, the internet was not the best place to convert my prospects into customers, so I decided to create a live funnel.

How could I get in front of members of my target market and convince them that I was the real deal?

I decided to create a one-hour workshop showing women how to repair a broken metabolism, and how to trigger weight loss and energy production in 30 days or less. I promised that this live workshop would give them every key they needed to make real change happen in their life.

I also showed a before/after photo from a woman I worked with in my dry-run training who is still a client, by the way. I knew I would have a lot of sign-ups and many wouldn't show, as is always the case with workshops. So I included a barrier to the process and pre-qualified my market by making prospects reserve their seat for $10.

I let them know that the fee would be returned in cash at the door when they showed up and it was just to reduce the no-show rate. I told them I wanted serious action-takers only. During this time, I had a few test-clients post that I was, in fact legit and that this workshop was a game-changer.

Then I targeted my market using special techniques to hone in on the avatar I described. Within a few days and about $40 in ad spend, I had booked my workshop.

The workshop was the lead magnet. My conversion rate was huge and I could easily scale this in the future. But right now I wanted to focus on slow steady growth since I was new in town. Since completing our last funnel, referral rates have been outstanding and we have not advertised or completed a workshop this month. Still, we are doing about five consults per week with almost 100% conversion to private personal training.

I also have an infant and I love spending time with her and my wife, so I don't want to scale up yet. I think the real beauty of this launch formula is that it is truly timeless. I want to enjoy the winter and ski on Tuesdays and Thursdays. I want to work on projects for my other businesses on the weekends and spend time with my family. It is comforting to know that at any time I can pull the trigger on my ads and book a workshop solid in just a few days.

The workshop leads to a special VIP tripwire funnel that I make available to members of my coaching program. But in short, my tripwire is a 1-on-1 strategy session I have taught my trainers how to complete and it has a 90%-100% conversion rate.

Everything is laid out for them, and I can teach it to anyone in a few hours. It takes about three practice sessions and it's a done deal. I have two trainers using it now with the exact same conversion rate of 90%-100%.

My workshop is converting at right around 75% and I have found that those that attend and don't sign up usually come back within a few weeks for a consult. I have also found that the ones who don't take the tripwire offer and meet with us for a 1-on-1 VIP consult, often send their friends in for a consult or to inquire when our next workshop will be. This means that the lead magnet itself is creating massive reciprocity.

I am a simple guy and I love having a simple life. I have downsized so much in the last few years. I now own and manage two fitness facilities, a software company, a small information products business and a worldwide coaching program that has reached 26 countries, believe it or not.

I am an engineer by nature and not a fitness trainer. I engineer fitness systems; I engineer fitness funnels; I engineer business models; I engineer experience. I recently realized that I love my clients and the relationships I have created with them, but I don't love counting reps. I don't love anything that I have already done before. I crave new experience and new ways of optimizing the lives of my training clients, business customers and business coaching students.

I love working 40 hours a week and I love the continuous variation that each week holds. That is why I have created multiple companies and business ventures. I am always looking for new ways to reengineer old ideas and make them better.

The funnel I outlined above is so simple to use, and it works like a finely tuned machine. I'm training my employees to give the workshop now so I can remove myself from the equation. If my conversion rate goes down after this, I will simply find another way to increase the conversion.

It is so comforting to know that I have funnels that consistently and predictably work. They work on both ends. My customers love the engineered journey, and my family loves the predictable nature of our income. I have used this soft launch technique across many markets including an information product business, a video coaching program, four brick-and-mortar fitness businesses, and two chiropractic offices, all with equal conversion rates and levels of success.

I'm 42 years old. I'm in decent shape and I have a nice bedside manner. That's it! If I can come into a town where I know nobody and launch a business in this way, surely you (probably having at least a dozen clients who already love you) can do the same or better.

This game is really quite simple when you know your conversion rates across every stage of your funnel. It is also easy when you know how to drive traffic to those funnels. When we know predictable outcomes, we can take predictable risks. I love predictable risk. You will too!

OK, once you have completed your soft launch, you will want to do a final inspection of the process and assess these areas.

- Conversion rate across your lead magnet
- Conversion rate across your tripwire
- Conversion rate across your core offer
- Overall funnel conversion rate
- Retention rate after conversion to core offer (Do your customers stay?)
- Ascension rate following consumption of core offer (Do your customers want more?)

After we have solid measurements on the above analytics, we will need to determine if we need to tweak any stage of the funnel to optimize the results for a re-launch or grand opening.

The next chapter will outline a collection of personal experiences with multiple grand openings across different niches. We will dive into the necessary steps used by event planners in all business niches to make sure grand openings go off with a bang and bring the customers.

CHAPTER ELEVEN

Your Grand Opening

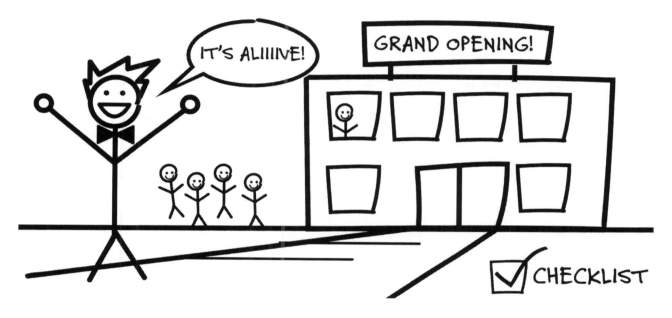

Congratulations! You made it to the last phase and few owners ever do. But if you are serious about having an awesome and eventful grand opening for your business, this chapter won't disappoint. We are going to cover all the intricate little details that you will need to remember when having your grand opening.

Before we get into it, I am going to make a few assumptions:

✓ — You have your business dialed in and you have completed all chapters of this book.

✓ — You have an actual brick-and-mortar location and your building is finished and ready to go.

✓ — You have staff. Having a grand opening as a one-man show is not only difficult but it will drain you for weeks.

Most grand openings are actual grand re-openings. I personally do not recommend having a grand opening unless you have been open for a few months. The planning and execution process for a grand opening is at minimum three months. You need to have a bulletproof plan to make this worth the investment.

As stated in the previous chapter, a grand opening is usually not necessary, but can be a very powerful customer acquisition tool, setting you apart from other businesses in your market if done correctly. If this phase is completed in error or haste, it will only serve to tell the public at large that you are disorganized and ineffective.

Grand Openings Do Require Capital

As with any marketing expense, you are expecting a positive return on your investment and grand openings are no exception. A typical grand opening will cost thousands. But if done effectively, will generate thousands in customer-acquisition and exposure dollars.

You can even look at a grand opening as a self-liquidating offer. If you break even on your grand opening, you are doing great, because you acquired new customers and gained exposure at a zero cost investment.

Below is a quick outline of everything you need to successfully plan and execute your big grand opening with laser precision.

Your Budget and Your Plan

How much do you have to spend? What do you want to do? These will dictate the level of financial investment required. Start with the day. What do you want to do every hour on the hour until the event is over to create the ultimate experience for your prospect?

The Flow and Activities of The Day

As stated above, you will need to know how you want your attendees to digest the experience. I recommend starting around 11 a.m. with a live event such as a speech, guest appearance or class to kick off the affair. Then you will need to move the prospects through your labyrinth of activities and sales funnels. That's what a grand opening is. It is a sales funnel that accomplishes two things.

First, a grand opening creates buyers through likability, trust and familiarity, promoting your best low-barrier offers. Second, it promotes relationships and exposes your brand, your story and your dedication to your market. Spend time architecting your experience, because this is where the money is made and the relationships are formed. You did not start a business just to make money, so make sure that you focus on all elements of your brand such as education, engagement, presence and altruism. Do not use this event as a blatant pitch fest. You have to blend your business needs with your need for community and giving back. Remember, help first, profit second.

Rain Date Planned

This is important, and if your event is outdoors and your activities are in a parking lot, make sure that they are covered against the elements, or that a rain location/date is scheduled. This is difficult, so I recommend having your grand opening in a weatherproof location.

Special Permits or Licenses

Depending on where you live and the zoning associated with your business, you may need special permitting to hold a grand opening. Find out what licenses or permits you will need to have your grand opening here: https://www.sba.gov/licenses-and-permits.

Get A Photographer

You need the pictures for Facebook Fan page images. OK, I highly recommend you hire a local photographer to cover your event with specific instructions to capture the right kind of images. You need images you can use for advertising, so make sure that the images make your business look popular, fun, easy to access and awesome. Make sure that customers are OK with being photographed. If someone complains, delete those images.

Red Carpet and Backdrop for Before Photos

I highly recommend advertising that you will be doing celebrity photo shoots and even have a local celebrity on hand who is willing to be photographed with all your prospects against a backdrop that features your logo. Set up the backdrop just like a Hollywood red carpet backdrop. Red carpets are cheap to rent and you can get a backdrop for $100 online. The pictures will be priceless, and you can collect emails to send the pictures to attendees. It's a killer lead generation strategy. Who is going to complain about you sending them celebrity photo shoot pics? Make sure you advertise the celebrity photo shoot in your marketing materials for the event.

Make Sure You Have Enough Parking

Super important and self-explanatory. If attendees cannot park, you will need to provide a shuttle service or rent nearby parking. Hopefully you have enough parking and this won't be an issue. If parking is an issue, I recommend a select invitee list of strategic attendees that allows you to use the opening as more of a networking event with the "who's who" of your local area.

Food and Catering

The fastest way to a person's heart is through their stomach and the food does not have to be expensive. Serve organic hot dogs, burgers, soda, water and beer and you will be fine.

Activities and Games

Highly recommended. If you are going to keep attendees in your target market at your event, you will need games and activities they can enjoy. These do not have to be expensive. You could have a plank contest to win T-shirts, or a Push-up contest to win an iPad or something. Think about what your market and their families would like to do and then scale it up or down according to your budget.

Prizes and Raffles

Always have a raffle so you can collect emails, phone numbers and addresses. You can use these to market after the event. Give away something in the $200 to $1,000 range and make it something everyone would like and could re-sell if they did not like it. An iPad or one-year transferable membership to your facility are two extreme ideas that would work great.

Live Entertainment

Not mandatory, but definitely a great idea. I recommend contacting a local band and offering them training in exchange for performing. All musicians need to have a solid public image and training will help that.

Speaker

This is completely optional and will vary in effectiveness depending on your area. A local college town will embrace a speaker and a rural town probably won't. You decide and plan accordingly.

Joint Venture or Strategic Partners

This is controversial, so I will throw out the idea and you run with it. If you have strategic partnerships in place for your efforts in the first seven phases of this launch sequence, then I can honestly say it can't hurt and you could actually share costs with your partners. For instance, if you had a local chiropractor and natural foods specialist at your grand opening giving scans and free protein shakes, this would create more draw but it would definitely dilute your marketing message at the time.

However, if your attendee chose chiropractic instead of fitness as their immediate solution, you would hope that your strategic partner would refer to you at a later date. I refer to this as the echo effect in marketing. The patient will remember going to your event and meeting the chiropractor and choose you over your competition when it comes to their fitness provider.

Signage

This is important. You need signage to have a grand opening. You need all sorts of signage to do it effectively. I recommend starting with vinyl banners and yard signs and moving up from there. Place yard signs at popular intersections and vinyl banners at your location. You can even rent temporary billboard space if you have highways near your facility with empty signs. These are very effective for grand openings, but cost money, so be prepared to pay for it. Remember, you are always buying your customers. If you have a good conversion system, you should not be afraid to pay money to acquire new clients.

Staffing

Please don't even think about holding a grand opening without staff. If you do you will soon regret it. First of all, grand openings work, which means you will have too many customers to handle effectively on your own. Secondly, you will burn yourself out trying to do everything *and* run a business. Customers who have a bad experience at the grand opening event may never fully trust you, nor become clients of your business in the future.

Invitee List

This depends on the size of your opening, but start with big names in your community and make sure you send the invitations months in advance. You could invite the mayor, fire department, the press, local business owners and their employees. If they RSVP that they will be in attendance you know you can push the advertising a little harder.

Tour Schedule

At your grand opening I highly recommend giving tours and having mock classes available for attendees to take at hourly intervals. You could do a tour one hour and a class the following hour and assessments the following hour, repeating the process throughout the day. That way, if your attendees show interest, you can escalate their experience while keeping their families entertained with food, games and activities.

Lead Magnets

Remember, your grand opening is a funnel and all your lead magnets need to be present at your grand opening. For instance, if one of your lead magnets is a downloadable Body Transformation Checklist, then you will need printed copies of this lead magnet available at your opening. Just like your online funnel, try to set up the lead magnet as an attractive giveaway that attendees get when they register for your drawing or raffle. In other words, you trade the checklist for an email. Your physical lead magnet should lead to the same conversion process you use with your online lead magnets.

Embedded Calls to Action

Try to have a definite embedded call to action involved in all the activities and events going on during your grand opening. Lead your prospect to the mouth of your conversion funnel or to consume one of your lead magnets through strategic conversations, planned events and activities. This process is what separates the pros from the amateurs when planning events. Look at any live event you have ever attended that revolved around growing a business. The live event was nothing more than a funnel to deliver value, create a relationship with you, and lead you to high-ticket investments or other lead magnets and splintered offers.

Swag

Swag items are just little trinkets you can give away that have your name on them. I have seen water bottles, pens, key chains and bracelets work well. When ordering swag, think about the needs of adults, businesses and kids, so you have a well-rounded arsenal of affordable swag. T-shirts and clothing do not make good swag items because they are cost-prohibitive. As a rule of thumb, try to keep swag items under $2 per item and order a limited quantity. When they are gone, they are gone. But you can always give them a lead magnet. Here is a million-dollar idea for you. Put the website address of your lead magnet squeeze page on your swag and not your company website. Put analytics on that squeeze page and take note of your hits.

Here is an example of a swag item done well. A water bottle that has your company name and this tag line: "Learn how much water you have to consume before your body is even able to burn fat." Go to Water2BurnFat.com to find out. This website address is set up with a squeeze page that offers a branded video showing five conditions you must meet before your body will burn fat. The video they receive will not only give them these answers, but also offer them an initial body composition analysis with your company.

Written Itinerary

You will need a schedule of events posted at your grand opening so attendees know what to expect throughout the day. Try to keep the best events for last, like finding out who wins the grand prize. This may keep your attendees there longer or make them come back to consume whatever late-day goodies you have planned. Make the entire day enjoyable and make sure the itinerary is packed.

Promotional Literature

See that the promotional literature you have created is present at your event in limited quantities. Make sure your flyers and gift cards are visible in multiple locations throughout your facility or event location.

The action items above will help make your grand opening profitable and memorable for your attendees. I have included a checklist below that you can use when creating your budget.

Here are some attractive items you could have at the site of your grand opening. Some are easy to procure and others will take connections, but these have been used successfully across multiple niches to make grand openings special

- Fire Truck
- Ambulance
- Police Car
- Race Car
- Helicopter
- Search lights
- Inflatable Wavy Guy
- Bounce House
- Giant Banners
- Balloons

Here are some ideas for food and drink depending on local regulations:

- Barbecue
- Finger foods
- Drink variety: water, juice, healthy shakes, organic wines.

You will want to provide some form of entertainment to anchor the experience. Here are some ideas for entertainment. Some are expensive while others may be free.

- Grand prize raffles
- Cool door prizes
- Random and hourly giveaways
- Celebrity or government official ribbon cutting
- Fitness games
- Tours
- After Party
- Short educational class
- Local charity event
- Fireworks and fire truck
- Local celebrities or athletes

- Photographer
- Videographer
- Acrobatic entertainers
- Balloon guys
- Face painting
- Magician
- Comedian
- Local band
- Local marching band
- Local dance group
- DJ

You should have activities planned for all ages at your grand opening. Here are some ideas you can use to keep people having fun and enjoying the experience.

Marketing your event is a process all by itself. Here are some quick ideas you can use to let your local community know you are coming in a big way.

Online Marketing

This is how to get the word out online that you are coming.

1 **Facebook Promoted Posts:** Use your fan page to target your market through strategically promoted posts.

- Make a post on your fan page
- Boost the post
- Target your audience
- Drive traffic to your "coming soon" page or grand opening page

2 **Organic SEO:** Optimize your "coming soon" page with your company name grand opening.

3 **Google AdWords:** Run ads for your business and target local keywords customers would use to find you. Here are some quick keyword examples that I have used:

- Personal Trainer [Your City]
- Weight Loss [Your City]
- [Your Company Name]
- Boot Camp [Your City]
- [Your Company Name] Grand Opening

> I have some resources on the FitProEvolution.com/Resources page of my website. These are tested resources that I have personally used with positive results.

Offline Marketing

The marketing you do that drives traffic using local resources.

1 **Direct Mail:** This is the easiest way to get news of your grand opening to your target market. Simply create a postcard and choose your targeting by area or zip code and mail. Most companies do direct mail notifications with postcards and oversized postcards as a standard. Make sure your postcard has an "a-offer/b-offer" design.

- **A-offer:** Your core message: You are having a grand opening
- **B-offer:** Drives them to a squeeze page to get an itinerary, checklist, price sheet etc

2 **Local Newspapers and Magazines:** See what the local newspaper charges for advertorials. This is a great way to get your core message to your target market and warm them up to you and your brand before the grand opening. A great way to do this is with an advertorial about you, your family and your message to the world through your brand. This story includes:

- Who you are and what you do
- Your story of struggle
- Your story of finding the solution
- The old way people would go about getting in shape and why it doesn't work
- The new way that you developed and the framework surrounding your brand
- Your story of creating your business and your "why"
- Invitation to your grand opening event

3 **Radio and Television:** Radio and television work in a similar and more expensive way than your local newspaper. Most people use radio and TV to get the word out about their grand opening and usually get the radio station to cover it. I have never used radio or television for any launch, so I cannot personally speak to its effectiveness. But some people use it with massive success.

4 **Press Releases and Media Releases:** I recommend using these with every launch and grand opening you do. They are extremely effective in getting the word out to the press and media about your business or event. I advise having these professionally written.

I have listed the sources I use for press release creation and submissions on my resources page at FitProEvolution.com/Resources

Feel free to check out all my tools for fitness launch success there.

You can also check out my area-exclusive video coaching program called Fitness Launch Academy at FitnessLaunchAcademy.com.

This program is designed to speed up and automate your ability to implement the core principles covered in this book.

Now you know how to hold a grand opening for your business. You have a checklist of items to include and some great strategies covering your end game, which is to acquire customers out of thin air.

This is a process and it takes practice. Even if you only follow this process 85% of the way through, you will avoid thousands of dollars in lost revenue, time-consuming headaches and potentially turning off your prospects before you even get a chance to meet them in person.

Openings are a science and I recommend that you be in business at least three months before you start to plan your grand opening. You can keep doing targeted soft launches and build up your customer base for months before you will really need to do something on a bigger scale.

Take it slow and easy. As long as you are breaking even and taking home enough to live on, all urgency is imagined. You are in such a good place to be able to slowly and strategically build your customer base with people you love working with.

I used to take whoever would give me money. Now I turn down people who do not fit my market or my long-term vision.

CHAPTER 12

Conclusion

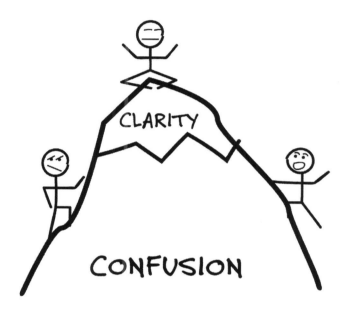

Thank you so much for going on this journey with me. I hope you had just as much fun and as many inspiring moments reading this book as I did when I wrote it. I have coached hundreds of fitness professionals to live a better life, wake up happier, make more money and work less through my programs, blog and private mentoring.

I am confident that if you read and implement the strategies and game plan laid out for you in this book, you will fall in love with the business that you build. You just have to take the first step. Throw away everything inside you that says you can't do this, and find that one place in the center of your fear that still holds hope. Nurture that. Believe in it. Don't let naysayers and toxic relationships steal that hope. Guard it with your entire being.

You have a gift the world needs. I think that is why I felt so compelled to write this book. My gift was not discovered until I stopped listening to the advice of negative people and started listening to my hope. I hoped one day I would be financially independent. I hoped one day I would be respected and looked up to. I hoped that one day I would have a family of my own and a lifestyle designed from the dreams within me.

I did it and so can you. Trust your gift. Trust your voice. Trust your path and trust God to deliver everything you need to make it happen. Don't be afraid to do the work. The amount of action steps laid out in this book are many, but they are finite. I have done it six times in two different offline niches with great success.

The secret is in the process. It is in reversing the pyramid and placing all the emphasis in all the right places. Your foundation, blueprinting, numbers and groundwork are the most important parts. The build, the polish and the dry run are only going to be successful if the architecture of your actual business model is solid.

The number one thing most fitness pros think they need is better marketing and more clients. What they really need is a bulletproof architecture, tested conversion systems and complete funnels. If they had these things, they would never look at marketing and client-getting as the answer. They would see it as the byproduct of a well-designed business model.

It can take years to see the real truth surrounding your business, and unfortunately some people never will. They will get caught up in every shiny ball that crosses their field of vision and fail to ask themselves if it resonates with their brand, their mission, their product ladder etc. Don't let this happen to you. Don't get derailed from your dream. You were designed for this. That's why you are reading this book. There are some action steps and groundwork you need to follow to avoid pitfalls, but ultimately you need to know who you really are at a core level. This is hard for some people to access or even explore, because it may be a painful experience. Just try. It starts by asking yourself some of the compass questions below.

The first thing you need to do is spend time finding out who you are and what you love to do:

Take some time and ask yourself these nine business clarification questions:

- **?** — Of all the things I'm doing right now, what are my favorites?

- **?** — What projects or activities make me feel good?

- **?** — What activities cause me to feel stress?

- **?** — What activities feel natural and easy?

- **?** — What do I want to work on but somehow never find the time for?

- **?** — What are my priorities right now?

? — What should my priorities be?

? — What do I want to be remembered for 3, 5, 10 years from now?

? — Will my current activities give me the platform I need to have the impact I want to have?

Then you need to construct or reconstruct your business to be in alignment with your answers to the questions above. When you do this, and use this as your compass to build everything else around these answers, it becomes hard to fail. Decisions surrounding the work that follows will be easy if you stick to your compass.

Next, figure out who you really want to serve. Who do you want to talk to every day? Who do you want to write for? Who do you want to motivate and help? Who do you want to impact?

When you know who you really want to help, you won't tire or get bored serving them. You can build your offering around serving this market segment. When you are excited about serving your market, you will wake up with a ton of purpose and joy in your heart. This is essential for the longevity of your model because you are the engine that fuels it. Without your passion, your business won't prosper.

Next, you will need to make sure that the market you truly want a relationship with actually exists. Rarely will your market choice be uncommon. If this is the case, you will need to find a new way to serve that is still in alignment with your true desires and wiring.

After this has been tested, verified and you have a green light, you should architect your business model and build out all the ladders, funnels and conversion systems so that you attract and keep the person you really want a relationship with. You do this through your strategic offerings and your unique gifts.

Once you have your model built out on paper, you just build it in real life and watch it take shape in front of your eyes. This will take work and there will be many sleepless nights and minor setbacks. But the steps are finite and this thought should keep you moving forward to the end.

The final steps are just to polish your edges and clean up the rough spots. Then you invite a select few people to run through your system and you correct all the little problems they encounter and optimize the experience so they want to continue and remain your customer.

Take care of any changes or tweaks that you need to make and increase your offer to a larger and more targeted audience. Nine times out of ten, this will be extremely successful and you can continue to expand through the implementation of perpetual soft launches. If you want to make a bigger impact and you have been in business successfully for a few months, you can start to plan and execute the steps necessary to kick off your big grand opening.

That's it in a nutshell. I have done it six times and generated more than $3 million through strategic and deliberate architecture of my dream life. You can do the same.

It wasn't always like this for me though. Just a few years ago, my life was a wreck. On the outside I may have had people fooled. But on the inside I was broken, hopeless and never imagined that I would actually finish the book that I had set out to write years ago. I was living in a city that was almost 1,000 miles away from my family and what I truly love. I had built my dreams on sand, literally. I was living in Charleston, South Carolina and I wanted four seasons. I wanted to ski. I wanted to hike in the woods and see trees with leaves.

Some people still think I am crazy for leaving, but I am so happy I stuck to my internal compass and kept the faith that I could have a life built around the things that make me happy and bring me deep inner joy. Every morning I wake up and have a cup of coffee and look out the window of my mountaintop home. I get to see my daughter many times throughout the day. I have a beautiful wife who is truly my best friend, shares my beliefs and values, and loves me for my crazy ideas and projects.

She is actually the one who encouraged me to finish this book, and to draft and create the life that this book is designed to help you construct as well. I have always wanted to have a close knit group of friends who loved fitness, business and living an optimum life. I have always wanted to create a community of game-changers and life-bringers and build a place where we could all go for inspiration, guidance and share ideas in a non-competitive environment.

This book is Step 1 on your journey with me. It was designed to help you navigate out of the place you may be stuck in.

Maybe you have an amazing family and a business you absolutely love, but are just working too much to see the ones you love most.

Maybe you work in a gym and you have always wanted to open your own business, but never knew which step to take first or how to persevere through it all.

Maybe you have tried and failed and you are afraid to get back on the horse again. You have become cynical and think success is for everyone else, but just not for you.

Maybe you have a business and it's floundering or has become stagnant and you just need new energy. You need to find some inspiration or ideas to bring life back into your business.

If any of the above scenarios resonate with you, I want to extend to you a personal invitation to join my **Fitness Launch Academy** program. Together, I want to resurrect the dream I had long ago of developing a community of fitness professionals dedicated to one thing. I'm calling all game-changers and lifestyle architects. Here are the prerequisites:

- You must be a supportive and generous person. Cynics not invited
- You must be dedicated to architecting your life and helping others architect theirs
- You must be dedicated to architecting your business and optimizing your funnels
- You must be willing to collaborate and share ideas

That's it! If the above describes you, I personally invite you to join our community and, of course, my location exclusive coaching program.

 You can learn more about joining at FitnessLaunchAcademy.com.

My Final Thoughts for You

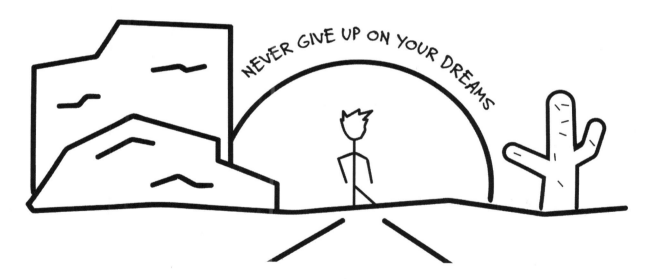

You are going to be successful. Plain and simple. Just wake up and say this to yourself every day. Settle for no other thought or belief. You will be amazed at what a change in your mindset will do for you.

Believe in your purpose. You were designed to be great, not good at something. It is your personal gift to the world. We all have one. You just have to find yours. It will happen when you start asking the right questions and stop worrying about what others expect of you.

For decades, I woke up worried about what people thought about me. I would battle internally on a daily basis and struggle with my value and my purpose. Days turned into weeks and weeks into years — then decades. I don't think I let go of worry, fear of failure, or fear of looking stupid until I was at least 35 years old. Almost immediately after I hit rock bottom and literally called out to God on my knees, my life started to clarify. My compass began to point north on a daily basis and I started making decisions in line with the questions I asked you above. I am not writing this to be evangelical. I do have my own spiritual beliefs and if you ask me I will share them with you. I am writing this to let you know that no matter where you are or how far you have fallen away from your true self or your big dream, you can always get back on course when you start asking the questions that lead you to your true self.

Never give up on your dreams. They will come to fruition if you keep them alive in your heart, believe they can be achieved, and take steps every day toward the direction of their realization. I am living proof that anyone can break the mold and go on to do great things. I believe in you and that is the sole purpose for writing this book. This is my message to you. Your gift will make room for you and bring you before many great and mighty things. Believe it!

CHAPTER 13

Resources/Next Steps

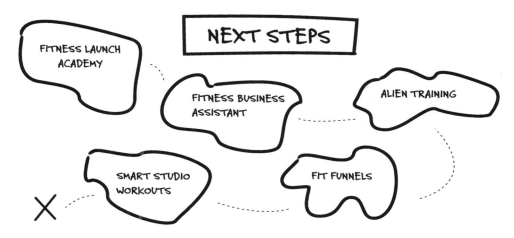

Here is a list of resources I have compiled to help you on your journey. Everything I develop, I pour my heart and soul into and I use all the tools below my website 365 days a year to increase client retention, streamline and automate my businesses, and coach my students.

FitProEvolution.com: Welcome to my new blog! I post fitness business strategies, tools and tips for productivity and ways to do more while working less.

FitProEvolution.com/Resources/: All the online tools and resources I use to organize my life, run my businesses, and simplify my life.

FitnessLaunchAcademy.com: I created this new area-exclusive coaching program to speed up and automate your success with implementing the core principles taught in my **Fitness Launch Formula** book. This program is the logical progression for anyone who loved my book and fulfills the above prerequisites.

FitnessBusinessAssistant.com: This is a revolutionary software platform I spent two years developing. It gives you the ability to create and deliver branded surveys, certificates, assessments, intake forms, messages, meal plans, cardio programs, education videos, special offers and more. FBA integrates with Mindbody software and allows you to sync client and financial data to your dashboard so you can track leads, customers, open rates, expenses, net profit and more.

AlienTraining.com: If you have ever wanted your own black book of cutting edge, outside-the-box exercise ideas you could easily plug into your current programming models, AlienTraining will not disappoint. It's packed with more than 300 hours of never-released videos showing you step-by-step how to double and triple your client retention with programming tweaks. These are the same training protocols I have used in all my facilities and are the driving force behind our high revenues and endless retention.

IdeaInception.com: My branding, identity, and publishing platform for fitness professionals. We help you design a killer brand, design and build your website and social media channels, build out your online and offline funnels, and integrate everything you need to take payments and make automated income.

The Fitness Entrepreneur's Choice for:

- Business Branding
- Website Development
- Information Product Development
- Graphic Design

- Book Publishing
- Sales Funnel Creation
- Custom Software Creation
- And More

Coming In 2016! Get On The Early Bird List

SmartStudioWorkouts.com

If you own a studio that offers private, small groups and group programs, you are going to fall in love with SSW. Nothing like this has ever been created. You will never have to think about or plan your programming again. This video vault and software combo will allow you to design world-class programs with periodization in seconds, not hours. Be sure to get on the early notification list today.

FitFunnels.com

Just as the name implies, Fit Funnels takes all the guesswork out of blueprinting, building, deploying and optimizing your fitness business acquisition and monetization funnels. This is a done-for-you funnel creation course that walks you step by step through 7 funnels you can build and deploy to automate your conversion process. This course comes complete with templates, checklists and training for all 7 funnels.

ABOUT THE AUTHOR

Brian Devlin lives in State College, PA, with his beautiful wife Kim and their precious daughter Charli. He walks to work every day and focuses on simplicity and essentialism in his day-to-day life. He co-created Fit Pro Evolution™ with his business partner and fellow entrepreneur Greg Crawford. Together Brian and Greg developed a powerful platform that helps thousands of fitness pros around the globe establish successful fitness businesses that impact the world. Brian's mission is to empower 10,000 fitness pros with the ability to use their unique gift to radically change the world around them, while living a life of prosperity and abundance for themselves.

You can learn more about Brian at his blog **www.FitProEvolution.com**.

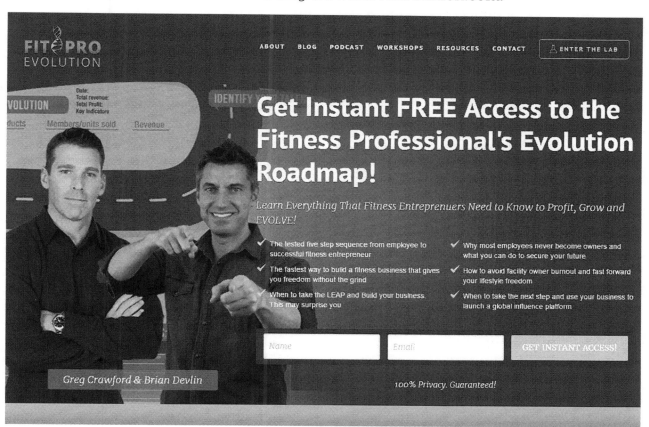

Be sure to get on Brian's mailing list so you can receive his time-saving tips, tricks and tactics designed to make your life as a fitness professional easier and more enjoyable.

Don't Forget Your 2 Invaluable
Free Bonus Videos and Start Up Cheat Sheet!

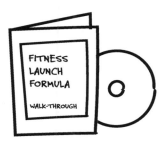

A personal walk-through video covering all the steps of the fitness launch formula

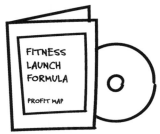

An in-depth and invaluable training video showing how to get your business to profit in month 1

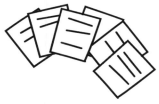

FITNESS LAUNCH FORMULA
CHEAT SHEETS

The fitness launch cheat sheets outlining all the steps of my formula

Congratulations, and thank you for investing in my book Fitness Launch Formula! Please don't forget to download your $297 bonus training package that I have included with your purchase.

This FREE training will really help you implement the strategies and tactics I discuss in the book quickly and efficiently. To grab your bonuses, simply go to www. FitProEvolution.com/flf-book-bonus/.

Just my way of saying "thank you" for investing in my book!

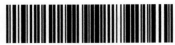

84014301R00109

Made in the USA
San Bernardino, CA
02 August 2018